KETO DIET MEAL PLAN
FOR WOMEN OVER 50

Ketogenic Cookbook for Easy Meal Planning.

28 Days of Low-Carb Recipes to
Boost Your Metabolism and Lose Weight.

Start a Healthy Lifestyle for a Happy Menopause

Elenore Jaslow

Copyright © 2021 by Elenore Jaslow

All rights reserved. The content contained within this book may not be reproduced, duplicated or transmitted without direct written permission from the author or the publisher.

Under no circumstances will any blame or legal responsibility be held against the publisher, or author, for any damages, reparation, or monetary loss due to the information contained within this book. Either directly or indirectly.

Legal Notice:

This book is copyright protected. This book is only for personal use. You cannot amend, distribute, sell, use, quote or paraphrase any part, or the content within this book, without the consent of the author or publisher.

Disclaimer Notice:

Please note the information contained within this document is for educational and entertainment purposes only. All effort has been executed to present accurate, up to date, and reliable, complete information. No warranties of any kind are declared or implied. Readers acknowledge that the author is not engaging in the rendering of legal, financial, medical or professional advice. The content within this book has been derived from various sources. Please consult a licensed professional before attempting any techniques outlined in this book.

By reading this document, the reader agrees that under no circumstances is the author responsible for any losses, direct or indirect, which are incurred as a result of the use of information contained within this document, including, but not limited to, – errors, omissions, or inaccuracies.

TABLE OF CONTENTS

INTRODUCTION 5

THE KETO BASICS 7

HORMONES AS YOU GET OLDER 10

HAVING A MEAL PLAN 12

DINING OUT 13

WEEK 1 17

   Monday - Day 1 17

   Tuesday - Day 2 21

   Wednesday - Day 3 24

   Thursday - Day 4 27

   Friday - Day 5 30

   Saturday - Day 6 34

   Sunday - Day 7 37

WEEK 2 40

   Monday - Day 8 40

   Tuesday - Day 9 44

   Wednesday - Day 10 47

   Thursday - Day 11 50

   Friday - Day 12 53

   Saturday - Day 13 57

   Sunday - Day 14 60

WEEK 3 63

   Monday - Day 15 63

   Tuesday - Day 16 66

   Wednesday - Day 17 69

   Thursday - Day 18 72

   Friday - Day 19 76

   Saturday - Day 20 79

   Sunday - Day 21 83

WEEK 4 87

   Monday - Day 22 87

   Tuesday - Day 23 91

   Wednesday - Day 24 95

   Thursday - Day 25 98

   Friday - Day 26 102

   Saturday - Day 27 106

   Sunday - Day 28 109

MEASUREMENT AND CONVERSIONS 114

CONCLUSION 115

INTRODUCTION

Women have likely experienced significant differences in how you must diet compared to how men can diet. They have a more challenging time losing weight because of their different hormones and how their bodies break down fats. Another factor to consider is your age group. As the body ages, it is essential to be more attentive to how you care for yourself. Aging bodies start to experience problems more quickly, which can be avoided with the proper diet and exercise plan. Keto works well for women of all ages, and this is because of how it communicates with the body. It will change the way that your body metabolizes, giving you a very personalized experience.

As we age, we naturally look for ways to hold onto our youth and energy. It's not uncommon to think about things that promote anti-aging. The great thing about the Keto diet is that it supports maximum health, from the inside out, working hard to ensure that you are in the best shape you can be.

For instance, indigestion becomes as common as you age. This happens because the body cannot break down certain foods as well as it used to. With all the additives and fillers, we all become used to putting our bodies through discomfort to digest regular meals. You will realize how your digestion will begin to change upon trying a Keto diet. You will no longer feel bloated or uncomfortable after you eat. If you notice this as a familiar feeling, you are likely not eating nutritious food enough to satisfy your needs and only result in excess calories.

Keto fills you up in all the ways you need, allowing your body to digest and metabolize all the nutrients truly. When you eat your meals, you should not feel the need to overeat to overcompensate for not having enough nutrients. Anything that takes the stress from any system in your body will become a form of anti-aging. You will quickly find this benefit once you start your Keto journey, as it is one of the first-reported changes that most participants notice. In addition to a healthier digestive system, you will also experience more regular bathroom usage, with little to none of the problems often associated with age.

While weight loss is one of the more common desires for most 50+ women who start a diet plan, the way that the weight is lost matters. If you have ever shed a lot of weight before, you have probably experienced the adverse effects of sagging or drooping skin that you were left to deal with. Keto rejuvenates the elasticity in your skin. You will be able to lose weight, and your skin will catch up. Instead of having to do copious amounts of exercise to firm up your skin, it should already be becoming firmer each day you are on the Keto diet. It is something that a lot of participants are pleasantly surprised to find out.

Women also commonly report a natural reduction in wrinkles and healthier skin and hair growth, in general. Many women who start the diet report that they notice reverse effects in their aging process. While the skin becomes healthier and suppler, it also becomes firmer. Even if you aren't presently losing weight, you will still be able to appreciate the effects that Keto brings to your skin and face. Your internal systems are becoming healthier and tend to show outside in a short amount of time. You will also begin to feel healthier. While it is possible to read about others' experiences, there is nothing like feeling this for yourself when you start Keto.

Everyone, especially women over 50, has day-to-day tasks draining and requires specific amounts of energy to complete. Aging can, unfortunately, take away from your energy reserve, even if you get enough sleep at night. It limits how you must live your life, which can become a very frustrating realization. Most diet plans bring about a stagnant feeling that you are supposed to get used to, but Keto does the exact opposite. Since your body is genuinely getting everything you need nutritionally; it will repay you with a sustained energy supply.

Another common complaint about women over 50 is that seemingly overnight, your blood sugar levels will be more sensitive than usual. While everyone must keep an eye on these levels, it is especially important for those in their 50s and beyond. High blood sugar can indicate that diabetes is on the way, but Keto can become a preventative measure. Additionally, naturally regulating elevated blood sugar levels also reduces systemic inflammation, which is also common for women over 50. You will notice that you have been feeling stiff lately, despite your efforts to exercise and stretch. This is likely due to a normal case of inflamed joints. Inflammation can also affect vital organs and is a precursor to cancer. Keto will support your path to an anti-inflammatory lifestyle.

Sugar is never great for us, but it turns out that sugar can become especially dangerous as we age. What is known as "sugar sag" can occur when you get older because the excess sugar molecules will attach themselves to the skin and protein in your body. It doesn't even necessarily happen because you are overeating sugar. Average sugar intake levels can also lead to this sagging as the sugar weakens the strength of your proteins that are supposed to hold you together. With sagging come even more wrinkles and arterial stiffening.

If you have any anti-aging concerns, the Keto diet will likely be able to address your worries. It is a diet that works extremely hard while allowing you to follow a relatively direct and straightforward guideline in return. While your motivation is necessary to form a successful relationship with Keto, you won't need to worry about doing anything "wrong" or accidentally breaking your diet. If you know how to give up your sugary foods and drinks while making sure that you consume the correct amount of carbs, you will be able to find success while on a diet.

As a woman over 50, you'll find that you will feel better, healthier, and younger, by implementing the simple steps that will tune your body into processing excess fats for energy. You'll build muscle, lose fat and look and feel younger.

THE KETO BASICS

Starting a new diet can seem overwhelming. If you are a beginner, I want to start off by telling you that you are in excellent hands. Whether you know about the ketogenic diet basics or nothing at all, you will learn everything you need to help you get started. Any time you have questions, feel free to use this book as your own personal guide. While it may seem like work at first, it will become easier with time. Soon enough, you won't need to look at the list of foods you can and cannot eat; it will just come naturally. For now, let's take a look at what exactly the ketogenic diet is and why it may work for you.

WHAT IS KETOSIS?

Ketosis may seem like a scary word, but it is a completely natural metabolic state your body will enter when there is no longer glucose for your body to run off of. Instead, your body will begin to use fat as fuel! Exciting, right? Once your body has limited access to blood sugar or glucose, your body will enter a state of ketosis. You see, as you consume a low-carb diet, the levels of insulin hormones in your body will decrease, and the fatty acids in your body will be released from the fat stores.

From this point, the fatty acids that are being released in your body are then transferred to your liver. Once in place, the fatty acids are then oxidized and turned into ketone bodies, which provide your body with energy. This process is important because the fatty acids cannot cross your blood-brain barrier, meaning it cannot provide energy to your brain (important).Once the process has occurred, ketones provide energy for your body and your brain, without ever needing glucose.

HOW TO KNOW YOU ARE IN KETOSIS

To understand whether you are in ketosis, you can take tests of urine or blood which will display a higher level of ketones in the body. But then, rather than depending on these tests, you can get a whole picture when you observe the following symptoms. They are:

INCREASED THIRST AND URINATION ALONG WITH DRY MOUT

When the diet changes to a low-carbohydrate one, it can cause water retention in the body. In a diet with a high amount of carbohydrates, the extra carbs are stored as glycogen in the liver. Glycogen is bound to water molecules.

So, when you shift to a low-carb diet, the amount of glycogen stored gets diminished, which in turn means you are storing less water and therefore a higher chance of dehydration. So there is a loss of excess fluid when you move to a high-fat diet and thus can make you feel thirstier. There would be increased urination also since electrolytes are also flushed out since the ketogenic diet is naturally diuretic.

KETO BREAT

Since ketone bodies called acetones escape through our breath, there is a possibility of making a person's breath smell fruity. The smell disappears in the long run. The ketone bodies can also escape through sweat.

KETOGENIC DIET FOR WOMEN

Choosing a diet that actually works for you can oftentimes seem like an impossible task. If you have tried diet after diet and you still keep failing, you are not alone! Your diet is key to your overall health. Before diving into any diet, it is vital to have all of the information. If you are a woman over fifty looking to turn your health around, the ketogenic diet may be perfect for you.

WHO CAN BENEFIT?

Before you begin any diet, you should always consult with your doctor to help start. This way, a professional will be able to help you track the changes in your body, and you will have a safe place to discuss your health and condition. In general, the ketogenic diet is beneficial for women who are:

- Not getting results from their current diet
- Binge constantly on high-carb foods
- Have issues with sex hormones
- Going through menopause

Before we go any further, it's important to know which foods are allowed and which foods are not allowed in the keto diet.

KETO APPROVED FOODS

- All natural plant and dairy fats – plant-based oils, ghee, butter, cheese and cream
- Dairy products, apart from milk (milk is not allowed because it contains high amounts of carbohydrates; however, when milk is broken down to process cheese, cream, yogurt or butter, the carbohydrates are broken down)
- Nut-based milk – coconut milk, almond milk, soy milk, hemp milk
- Low-carb vegetables – leafy greens, vegies that grow above ground, ginger, onions, garlic
- Low carb fruits – berries, kiwi
- Sugar-free chocolates and condiments
- Keto sugar substitutes

KETO NON-APPROVED FOODS

- Grains, beans, legumes, lentils, rice, oats, chickpeas, barley, wheat, corn, sorghum
- Tubers – potatoes, beets, squash, yams and other starchy veggies
- Animal milk
- High-carb fruits – apples, peaches, bananas, mangoes, pineapples, melons, etc.
- Grain flours, wheat flours, chickpea flour
- High carb processed foods.

It's important that you make a habit out of reading the nutritional labels of everything you buy for you to better control your carbohydrate intake. As a rule of thumb, always go with the natural option instead of the processed option. So, for example, instead of buying store-bought chicken broth, make your own broth at home or instead of buying processed almond milk, make your own. This way, you can control all the ingredients that go into it and avoid the preservatives used to increase the shelf life of the particular item.

HORMONES AS YOU GET OLDER

MENOPAUSE

The most common result of aging-related hormonal fluctuations is menopause. Around age 50, women's ovaries start producing decreasing quantities of progesterone and estrogen; the adrenal gland attempts to compensate by creating more follicle-stimulating hormone (FSH).

While menopause is normal and happens to most girls, a few of the signs can be bothersome or even harmful. Symptoms may include these:

- Hot flashes
- Vaginal dryness and atrophy resulting in painful intercourse
- Reduced libido
- Insomnia
- Irritability/melancholy
- Osteoporosis may increase the probability of bone fractures

Assist with Symptoms: for several decades, doctors prescribed long-term utilization of an oral estrogen/progesterone mix to relieve these symptoms.

However, a study in the early 2000s demonstrated that those taking hormone replacement therapy had a greater chance of stroke, cardiovascular disorder, breast cancer, and blood clots.

Present guidelines imply that it is fine to take progesterone and estrogen for a brief period to assist with the transition to menopause and there is ongoing research investigating the efficacy and safety of various progesterone and estrogen formulas that may possibly be utilized for longer amounts of time.

Alternative therapies, for example bioidentical hormones generated from animal or plant sources, have not yet been thoroughly assessed for safety and efficacy. So for today, try the listed below:

- Non-hormonal drugs can handle hot flashes
- Topical herbal lotion used vaginally can assist with painful sex.
- Leading a healthy lifestyle that incorporates a balanced diet, regular physical activity, and anxiety management help relieve many symptoms of menopause.

It is also important for women to have regular bone-density screenings starting at age 65 to capture osteoporosis early.

NOT-SO-TENACIOUS D

Called the sunshine vitamin, as your skin synthesizes it following exposure to the sun, vitamin D acts as a hormone to help maintain strong bones and also regulate your immune system in addition to your own muscle and nerve function. Research indicates that vitamin D might also play a part in shielding cognition: 65-or-older people, who have been deficient in vitamin D, had a 53 percent greater chance of developing dementia; due to the severely paralyzed, the risk increased by 125 percent. The capability to develop into deficient increases with age. As you get older, your skin becomes much less effective in utilizing the sun's beams to create vitamin D, which means that your body needs more.

Try this: think about a daily vitamin D supplement as you might be unable to get enough out of food and by exposure alone. While the girls in their 50s and 60s get 600 ius daily, that is probably not sufficient for everybody. In a small pilot study presented at the society for endocrinology's yearly meeting, individuals who obtained 2,000 ius per day for 2 weeks had reduced blood pressure, lower levels of the stress hormone cortisol, as well as far better fitness functionality compared to placebo takers. But do not exceed this amount. Some research has linked elevated doses to an increased chance of developing kidney stones.

CHANGE OF HEART

The prevalence of heart attack in women increases significantly as soon as they reach menopause. Estrogen helps keep blood vessels pliable, and its decrease might explain why blood pressure and LDL, or bad cholesterol, often grow in this time period. Additionally, late peri- and postmenopause are correlated with higher fat deposits around the center that has been associated with an increased risk (as much as 54 percent) of cardiovascular disease.

The fat that forms on your center is particularly poisonous: it generates compounds like inflammatory proteins called cytokines, which are associated with insulin resistance and type 2 diabetes in addition to heart disease. One possible solution would be to begin hormone treatment, but time might be crucial. Should you move on HT while you are experiencing perimenopause, it might help protect you from developing this larger belly. But should you wait till you have passed menopause, then it might be too late, if you cannot take HT or don't want to, concentrate on committing to regular exercise and eating a diet low in sugar and saturated fat and full of vegetables, fish, nuts, and lean protein.

HAVING A MEAL PLAN

When you have a complete meal plan laid out in front of you, you are in a better position to have an idea as to what your diet would look like in the days to come. If you have to spontaneously decide what you will prepare to eat every time you are in the kitchen, your chances of getting off the rails become pretty high.

You can start by first calculating how many calories you are going to consume a day.

The next step would be to decide which macronutrients will have to be incorporated and in what proportion for your body to reach that goal. Remember that the rule of thumb is 75, 20, 5: for fats, proteins, and carbs, respectively.

CALORIES AND LOSING WEIGHT

In the ketogenic diet or in any other diet regimen, you need to work your calories in order to maintain, gain, or lose weight.

Simply put, if you want to maintain weight, then you need to take in as many calories as you burn. If you want to gain weight, then you need to take in more calories than you burn. And finally, if you want to lose weight, you need to burn more calories than you take in.

Let's say that again: if you want to lose weight, then you need to burn more calories than you take in. That's the simplest formula, and it applies even in the ketogenic diet.

CALCULATING YOUR DAILY CALORIC INTAKE

Many people think that calculating your calories while you are on a keto diet is not very important, but it is always good to watch how many calories you consume a day. It would help if you calculated how many calories you get to consume every day by the idea of how much weight you want to lose.

If your body needs 2,000 calories a day, but you consume only 1,400, your body is in a caloric deficit, so it will have to tap into your body's fat reserves, and this will result in a loss of weight. There are various calculators available online that can be used to calculate your daily caloric intake taking into account your objectives, age, height, activity level, and other factors.

In general, if you want to lose weight, you need to subtract around 600 calories from your daily caloric needs. So less than 1,000-1,200 calories if you are a woman.

DINING OUT

When there is so much going on in your life, it might become difficult to stick to a diet. However, you should approach the keto diet with the mindset that you are making a lifestyle change, and not that you are looking for a quick fix by following the rules of a diet. When you change your mindset and begin to incorporate the diet into various aspects of your life, you will truly begin to appreciate what you are working towards and the health benefits that you can experience by maintaining your keto lifestyle.

Being on a keto diet does not mean that you can now never eat out again or go out with your friends and enjoy yourself. You should be able to have fun, enjoy good food, and do all of the things that you love to do, otherwise your diet will feel like a prison, and you will find yourself eating cheat meals more often and going back and forth between the keto diet and not seeing any changes. Below are a few tips that you can use to eat out with the keto diet.

PLAN AHEAD

Before you head out or order in, you should take a look and see if there are any keto restaurants or restaurants that offer keto-friendly food options that are near your location. You can check this using Google or Yelp, or by typing in the keyword "keto" when searching for food on any food ordering app. Restaurants that should have keto-friendly foods are burger restaurants, Mexican restaurants, places that sell breakfast and brunch options, and places that have salad bars.

You should also make sure that you take a look at each restaurant's menu to check if there are any meals or other food items that are either marked keto or sound like they could be keto friendly. Many restaurants have updated their menus to include this type of information to help their customers who have specific dietary requirements order food. You can also call the restaurant if you are unsure about anything or if you have any questions before you place your order online or go out.

ORDERING

If you do not have much of a choice and you are ordering in or eating out at a non-keto restaurant, then you will need to select your meals carefully when you are placing your order. You should take some time and go through each item on their menu if you were not able to do so before online.

When ordering non-keto foods, you should look at the food options that have little to no carbs included in the dish, or carbs that can be removed from the dish. You should choose a meal that includes some non-starchy vegetables like arugula, asparagus, bell peppers, broccoli, brussels sprouts, cauliflower, kale, mushrooms, spinach, and tomatoes, healthy fats like avocado, and a moderate amount of protein.

When checking through their menu, you should also be aware that there are some foods that are prepared in such a way that they include added sugar and carbohydrates while they are cooking the food. Some examples of how restaurants can include added sugar and carbohydrates into a dish include coating some foods with a non-keto-friendly breading, using croutons in salads, adding syrup or jam to dishes to give them a sweet flavor, using tomato sauce or paste to give some foods an extra tangy tomato taste, thickening sauces with flour, pouring gravy over a dish, serving a dish with dried fruit, and using potatoes in some dishes, like soup and stew.

If you remove starch from a meal, such as asking them to not include a potato bake in a meal, and you are now only left with protein and nonstarchy vegetables on your plate, you should consider adding a side that is high in fat, such as avocado or egg. You could also ask them to add some butter or olive oil that can go over your vegetables, if they do not have many sides that they can offer you that are high in fats.

Another thing you should check for before you order is for condiments and other sauces. Condiments and other sauces can have many added sugars contained in them. If possible, you can ask them what they made the sauce with, or if they can remove the sauce or put it separately and not mixed in or drizzled over the food. If you order steak, you should make sure that they do not cook it with a basting like BBQ sauce and ask them to season it using only salt, pepper, and whichever other keto-friendly spice that you like that they do not mind doing for you. Otherwise, you can ask them to cook it without any spices or sauces and add your own when it arrives at your table.

There are many beverages that you should avoid on the keto diet. One can never be sure what a restaurant or takeaway puts into their drinks, so you should try to avoid drinking most of their beverage options. Beverages that you can include when ordering are infused water with cucumber, lemon, or lime, soda water, sparkling water, water, and unsweetened tea and coffee. You should ensure that they do not give you milk with your tea or coffee or ask them if they can bring you some heavy cream instead.

If you cannot find any meals on their menu to your tastes or which are not keto-friendly, then you can order a few of their sides, such as a side salad, cooked vegetables, olives, a boiled egg, scrambled egg, bacon, an omelet, and so on. If you mix a few of the different sides that they offer together, you can make your own keto-friendly meal.

If you are ever unsure about what is in a specific meal or how the restaurant prepares certain foods, then you can always ask. Most restaurant employees are happy to give you a rundown of their foods, and sometimes if they are not too busy, they can prepare a more keto-friendly version of one of their meals for you. So, do not be afraid to ask them questions.

There are some wonderful keto-friendly dessert recipes out there. However, when you go to a non-keto restaurant, you will need to look for other alternatives, especially if your group wants to stay for dessert, or you are craving something sweet when ordering from home. You should try to avoid the restaurant's dessert menu and check if they have some other options. You may need to ask someone at the restaurant if they would mix some things together for you, but you can look through the menu as well. Some dessert ideas you could order include herbal tea, a cheese platter, dark chocolate, some berries served in cream, or a coffee with cream.

When I go out, I like to order a rump or sirloin steak with a side green salad or a side of cooked vegetables, such as spinach or any other non-starchy vegetable. If you order a side salad, then you should check to make sure you can eat all the vegetables that are included in the salad, especially if you have removed a few food items from the salad. Not all salads are the same depending on the restaurant you order from, but you can generally eat a green salad without worrying if it is keto friendly. Also, if you order a cooked vegetable side, you should ask how it is prepared to make sure that they do not include any added sugars or carbohydrates in the cooking process.

JUST IN CASE

When you have been doing the keto diet for a while, you will become more familiar with the restaurants in your area and whether they have any keto-friendly options or not. If you know that you might struggle to find something at a restaurant when you are meeting up with your friends, then you might need to eat something before you leave the house and then order a side that you can nibble on while your friends are eating. That way, you will not feel left out by your friends, nor will you be hungry.

In less formal situations, such as going for a picnic or hike with friends and family, or visiting your family for a Sunday lunch, you can prepare your own meals to take with you if they are fine with you doing this (which they should not have a problem with). By doing this, you do not need to rely on anyone preparing you a separate lunch that is keto-friendly when everyone else is eating something else.

WEEK 1

MONDAY - DAY 1 - BREAKFAST

LEMON & CUCUMBER JUICE

Preparation Time: 10 minutes

Cooking Time: 0 minutes

Servings: 2

INGREDIENTS:

- 2 large cucumbers, sliced
- 2 apples, cored and sliced
- 4 celery stalks
- 1 (1-inch) piece fresh ginger, peeled
- 1 lemon, peeled

DIRECTIONS:

1. Add all ingredients into a juicer and extract the juice according to the manufacturer's method.
2. Pour into 2 glasses and serve immediately.

NUTRITION:

Calories: 230; Fat: 2.1g; Protein: 1.2g; Carbohydrates: 1.3g.

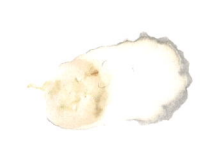

MONDAY - DAY 1 - LUNCH
KETO GROUND BEEF AND GREEN BEANS

Preparation Time: 5 minutes

Cooking Time: 10 minutes

Servings: 2

INGREDIENTS:

1 ½ ounce butter

8 ounces green beans, fresh, rinsed and trimmed

10 ounces ground beef

¼ cup crème fraîche or home-made mayonnaise, optional

Pepper and salt to taste

DIRECTIONS:

1. Over moderate heat in a large, frying pan; heat a generous dollop of butter until completely melted.
2. Increase the heat to high and immediately brown the ground beef until almost done, for 5 minutes. Sprinkle with pepper and salt to taste.
3. Decrease the heat to medium; add more butter and continue to fry the beans in the same pan with the meat for 5 more minutes, stirring frequently.
4. Season the beans with pepper and salt as well. Serve with the leftover butter and add in the optional crème fraiche or mayonnaise, if desired.

NUTRITION:

Calories: 513; Fat: 44g; Protein: 30g; Carbohydrates: 8.5g.

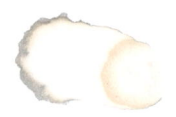

MONDAY - DAY 1 - DINNER
PASTA FREE LASAGNA

Preparation Time: 20 minutes

Cooking Time: 56 minutes

Servings: 12

INGREDIENTS:

2 large eggplants, cut into 1/8-inch thick slices lengthwise

Salt, as required

1 large organic egg

15 ounces part-skim ricotta

½ cup plus 2 tablespoons Parmesan cheese, grated and divided

4 cups sugar-free tomato sauce

16 ounces part-skim mozzarella cheese, shredded

2 tablespoons fresh parsley, chopped

DIRECTIONS:

1. Preheat the oven to 375°F.
2. Arrange the eggplant slices onto a smooth surface in a single layer and sprinkle with salt.
3. Set aside for about 10 minutes.
4. With a paper towel, pat dry the eggplant slices to remove the excess moisture and salt.
5. Heat a greased grill pan over medium heat and cook the eggplant slices for about 3 minutes per side.
6. Remove the eggplant slices from the grill pan and set aside.
7. In a medium bowl, place the egg, ricotta cheese and ½ cup of Parmesan cheese and mix well.
8. In the bottom of a 9x12-inch casserole dish, spread some tomato sauce evenly.
9. Place 5-6 eggplant slices on top of the sauce.

10. Spread some of the cheese mixture over eggplant slices and top with some of the mozzarella cheese.

11. Repeat the layers and sprinkle with the remaining Parmesan cheese.

12. Cover the casserole dish and bake for about 40 minutes.

13. Uncover the baking dish and bake for about 10 more minutes.

14. Remove the baking dish from oven and set aside for about 5-10 minutes before serving.

15. Cut into 12 equal-sized portions and serve, garnishing with fresh parsley.

NUTRITION:

Calories: 200; Fat: 1g; Protein: 18.2g; Carbohydrates: 8g.

TUESDAY - DAY 2 - BREAKFAST
MORNING COCONUT PORRIDGE

Preparation Time: 1 minute

Cooking Time: 5 minutes

Servings: 1

INGREDIENTS:

- 1 egg, beaten
- 1 tablespoon coconut milk
- 2 tablespoons coconut flour
- 2 teaspoons butter
- 1 cup water
- 1 pinch salt
- 2 tablespoons flax seeds
- Blueberries and raspberries

DIRECTIONS:

1. Put the flax seeds, coconut flour, water, and salt into a saucepan.
2. Heat this mixture until it has thickened slightly
3. Remove the mixture from the heat. Add beaten egg and put it on the stove again. Whisk slowly until you get a creamy texture.
4. Remove from the heat, add the butter and stir.
5. Serve with coconut milk, blueberries, and raspberries.

NUTRITION:

Calories 486; Fat 27g; Protein; 15g; Carbohydrates 6g.

TUESDAY - DAY 2 - LUNCH
CHEESY TILAPIA

Preparation Time: 10 minutes

Cooking Time: 10 minutes

Servings: 8

INGREDIENTS:

- 2 pounds tilapia fillets
- ½ cup Parmesan cheese, grated
- 3 tablespoons mayonnaise
- ¼ cup unsalted butter, softened
- 2 tablespoons fresh lemon juice
- ¼ teaspoon dried thyme, crushed
- Salt and ground black pepper, to taste

DIRECTIONS:

1. Preheat the broiler of the oven.
2. Grease a broiler pan.
3. In a large bowl, mix together all ingredients except tilapia fillets. Set aside.
4. Place the fillets onto the prepared broiler pan in a single layer.
5. Broil the fillets for about 2-3 minutes.
6. Remove the broiler pan from the oven and top the fillets with cheese mixture evenly.
7. Broil for about 2 minutes further.
8. Serve hot.

NUTRITION:

Calories: 185; Fat: 9.8g; Protein: 23.2g; Carbohydrates: 1.4g.

TUESDAY - DAY 2 - DINNER
PAPRIKA CHICKEN

Preparation Time: 10 minutes

Cooking Time: 35 minutes

Servings: 4

INGREDIENTS:

4 chicken breasts, skinless and boneless, cut into chunks

2 tablespoons paprika

2 ½ tablespoons olive oil

1 ½ teaspoons garlic, minced

2 tablespoons fresh lemon juice

Pepper

Salt

DIRECTIONS:

1. Preheat the oven to 350°F.
2. In a small bowl, mix together garlic, lemon juice, paprika, and olive oil.
3. Season chicken with pepper and salt.
4. Spread 1/3 bowl mixture on the bottom of the casserole dish.
5. Add chicken into the casserole dish and rub with dish sauce.
6. Pour remaining sauce over chicken and rub well.
7. Bake for 30-35 minutes.
8. Serve and enjoy.

NUTRITION:

Calories: 380; Fat: 22g; Protein: 14g; Carbohydrates: 2.6g.

WEDNESDAY - DAY 3 - BREAKFAST
BREAKFAST ROLL-UPS

Preparation Time: 5 Minutes

Cooking Time: 15 Minutes

Servings: 5 roll-ups

INGREDIENTS:

- Non-stick cooking spray
- 10 slices cooked bacon
- 1½ cups cheddar cheese, shredded
- Pepper and salt
- 10 large eggs

DIRECTIONS:

1. Preheat a skillet on medium to high heat, then combine two of the eggs in a mixing bowl using a whisk.
2. After the pan has become hot, lower the heat to medium-low heat, then put in the eggs. If you want to, you can use some cooking spray.
3. Season eggs with some pepper and salt.
4. Cover the eggs and leave them to cook for a couple of minutes or until the eggs are almost cooked.
5. Drizzle around 1/3 cup of cheese on top of the eggs, then place 2 strips of bacon.
6. Roll the egg carefully on top of the fillings. The roll-up will almost look like a taquito. If you have a hard time folding over the egg, use a spatula to keep the egg intact until the egg has molded into a roll-up.
7. Put aside the roll-up, then repeat the above steps until you have four more roll-ups; you should have 5 roll-ups in total.

NUTRITION:

Calories: 412.2; Fat: 31.66g; Protein: 28,21g; Carbohydrates: 2.26g.

WEDNESDAY - DAY 3 - LUNCH
CAULIFLOWER AND CASHEW NUT SALAD

Preparation Time: 10 Minutes

Cooking Time: 5 Minutes

Servings: 4

INGREDIENTS:

1 head cauliflower, cut into florets

½ cup black olives, pitted and chopped

1 cup roasted bell peppers, chopped

1 red onion, sliced

½ cup cashew nuts

Chopped celery leaves, for garnish

For the dressing:

Olive oil

Mustard

Vinegar

Salt and pepper

DIRECTIONS:

1. Add the cauliflower into a pot of boiling salted water. Allow to boil for 4 to 5 minutes until fork-tender but still crisp.
2. Remove from the heat and drain on paper towels, then transfer the cauliflower to a bowl.
3. Add the olives, bell pepper, and red onion. Stir well.
4. Make the dressing: In a separate bowl, mix the olive oil, mustard, vinegar, salt, and pepper. Pour the dressing over the veggies and toss to combine.
5. Serve topped with cashew nuts and celery leaves.

NUTRITION:

Calories: 298; Fat: 20g; Protein: 8g; Carbohydrates: 4g.

WEDNESDAY - DAY 3 - DINNER
GARLICKY PRIME RIB ROAST

Preparation Time: 15 minutes

Cooking Time: 1 hour 35 minutes

Servings: 15

INGREDIENTS:

- 10 garlic cloves
- 2 teaspoons dried thyme
- 2 tablespoons olive oil
- Salt
- Ground black pepper
- 1 grass-fed prime rib roast

DIRECTIONS:

1. Mix the garlic, thyme, oil, salt, and black pepper. Marinate the rib roast with garlic mixture for 1 hour.
2. Warm-up oven to 500°F.
3. Roast for 20 minutes. Lower to 325°F and roast for 65-75 minutes.
4. Remove, then cool down for 10-15 minutes, slice, and serve.

NUTRITION:

Calories: 499; Fat: 25.9g; Protein: 61.5g; Carbohydrates: 0.7g.

THURSDAY - DAY 4 - BREAKFAST
BRACING GINGER SMOOTHIE

Preparation Time: 5 minutes

Cooking Time: 5 minutes.

Servings: 2

INGREDIENTS:

⅓ cup coconut cream

⅔ cup water

2 tablespoons lime juice

1 ounce spinach, frozen

2 tablespoons ginger, grated

DIRECTIONS:

1. Blend all the ingredients. Add 1 tablespoon lime at first and increase the amount if necessary.
2. Top with grated ginger and enjoy your smoothie!

NUTRITION:

Calories: 82; Fat: 8g; Protein: 1g; Carbohydrates: 3g.

THURSDAY - DAY 4 - LUNCH
CHICKEN AVOCADO SALAD

Preparation Time: 10 minutes

Cooking Time: 10 minutes

Servings: 3

INGREDIENTS:

- 2 chicken breasts, cooked and cubed
- 1 tablespoon fresh lime juice
- 2 avocados, peeled and pitted
- 2 Serrano chili peppers, chopped
- ¼ cup celery, chopped
- 1 onion, chopped
- 1 cup cilantro, chopped
- 1 teaspoon kosher salt

DIRECTIONS:

1. Scoop out the pulp from the avocados and place it in the bowl.
2. Mash the avocado flesh using a fork.
3. Add remaining ingredients and mix until well combined.
4. Serve and enjoy.

NUTRITION:

Calories: 236; Fat: 10.6g; Protein: 29g; Carbohydrates: 4.5g.

THURSDAY - DAY 4 - DINNER
EGG DROP SOUP

Preparation Time: 5 minutes

Cooking Time: 15 minutes

Servings: 2

INGREDIENTS:

- 3 cups chicken broth
- 2 cups Swiss chard chopped
- 2 eggs, whisked
- 1 teaspoon grated ginger
- 1 teaspoon ground oregano
- 2 tablespoons coconut aminos
- Salt and pepper

DIRECTIONS:

1. Heat your broth in a saucepan.
2. Slowly drizzle in the eggs while stirring slowly.
3. Add the Swiss chard, grated ginger, oregano, and the coconut aminos. Next, season it and let it cook for 5-10 minutes.

NUTRITION:

Calories: 225; Fat: 19g; Protein: 11g; Carbohydrates: 4g.

FRIDAY - DAY 5 - BREAKFAST
BACON CHEESEBURGER WAFFLES

Preparation Time: 10 Minutes

Cooking Time: 20 Minutes

Servings: 4

INGREDIENTS:

Toppings

Pepper and salt to taste

1 ½ ounces cheddar cheese

4 tablespoons sugar-free barbecue sauce

4 slices bacon

4 ounces ground beef, 70% lean meat and 30% Fat

Waffle dough

Pepper and salt to taste

3 tablespoons parmesan cheese, grated

4 tablespoons almond flour

¼ teaspoon onion powder

¼ teaspoon garlic powder

1 cup cauliflower crumbles

2 large eggs

1 ½ ounces cheddar cheese

DIRECTIONS:

1. Shred about 3 ounces of cheddar cheese, then add in cauliflower crumbles in a bowl and put in half of the cheddar cheese.

2. Put spices, almond flour, eggs, and parmesan cheese into the mixture, then mix and put aside for some time.

3. Thinly slice the bacon and cook in a skillet on medium to high heat.

4. After the bacon is partially cooked, put in the beef, cook until the mixture is well done.

5. Put the excess grease from the bacon mixture into the waffle mixture. Set aside the bacon mix.

6. Use an immersion blender to blend the waffle mix until it becomes a paste, then add half of the mix into the waffle iron and cook until it becomes crispy.

7. Repeat for the remaining waffle mixture.

8. As the waffles cook, add sugar-free barbecue sauce to the ground beef and bacon mixture in the skillet.

9. Then proceed to assemble waffles by topping them with half of the remaining cheddar cheese and half the beef mixture. Repeat this for the remaining waffles, broil for around 1-2 minutes until the cheese has melted, then serve right away.

NUTRITION:

Calories: 405; Fat: 33.9g; Protein: 18.8g; Carbohydrates: 4.4g.

FRIDAY - DAY 5 - LUNCH
SHRIMP STEW

Preparation Time: 15 minutes

Cooking Time: 20 minutes

Servings: 6

INGREDIENTS:

¼ cup olive oil

¼ cup onion, chopped

¼ cup roasted red pepper, chopped

1 garlic clove, minced

1 ½ pounds raw shrimp, peeled and deveined

1 (14-ounce) can sugar-free diced tomatoes with chilies

1 cup unsweetened coconut milk

2 tablespoons Sriracha

2 tablespoons fresh lime juice

Salt and ground black pepper, to taste

¼ cup fresh cilantro, chopped

DIRECTIONS:

1. In a wok, heat the oil over medium heat and sauté the onion for about 4–5 minutes.
2. Add the red pepper and garlic and sauté for about 4–5 minutes.
3. Add the shrimp and tomatoes and cook for about 3–4 minutes.
4. Stir in the coconut milk and Sriracha and cook for about 4–5 minutes.
5. Stir in the lime juice, salt and black pepper and remove from the heat.
6. Garnish with cilantro and serve hot.

NUTRITION:

Calories: 289; Fat: 16g; Protein: 27.1g; Carbohydrates: 7g.

FRIDAY - DAY 5 - DINNER
KETO RED CURRY

Preparation Time: 20 minutes

Cooking Time: 15-20 minutes

Servings: 6

INGREDIENTS:

- 1 cup broccoli florets
- 1 large handful of fresh spinach
- 4 tablespoons coconut oil
- ¼ medium onion
- 1 teaspoon garlic, minced
- 1 teaspoon fresh ginger, peeled and minced
- 2 teaspoons soy sauce
- 1 tablespoon red curry paste
- ½ cup coconut cream

DIRECTIONS:

1. Add half the coconut oil to a saucepan and heat over medium-high heat.
2. When the oil is hot, put the onion in the pan and sauté for 3-4 minutes, until it is semi-translucent.
3. Sauté garlic, stirring, just until fragrant, about 30 seconds.
4. Lower the heat to medium-low and add broccoli florets. Sauté, stirring, for about 1-2 minutes.
5. Now, add the red curry paste. Sauté until the paste is fragrant, then mix everything.
6. Add the spinach on top of the vegetable mixture. When the spinach begins to wilt, add the coconut cream and stir.
7. Add the rest of the coconut oil, the soy sauce, and the minced ginger. Bring to a simmer for 5-10 minutes.
8. Serve hot.

NUTRITION:

Calories: 265; Fat: 7.1g; Protein: 4.4g; Carbohydrates: 2.1g.

SATURDAY - DAY 6 - BREAKFAST
SESAME KETO BAGELS

Preparation Time: 10 minutes

Cooking Time: 15 minutes

Servings: 6

INGREDIENTS:

- 2 cups almond flour
- 3 eggs
- 1 tablespoon baking powder
- 2 ½ cups Mozzarella cheese, shredded
- ½ cream cheese, cubed
- 1 pinch salt
- 2-3 teaspoons sesame seeds

DIRECTIONS:

1. Preheat the oven to 425°F.
2. Use a medium bowl to whisk the almond flour and baking powder. Add the mozzarella cheese and cubed cream cheese into a large bowl, mix and microwave for 90 seconds. Place 2 eggs into the almond mixture and stir in thoroughly to form a dough.
3. Part your dough into 6 portions and make into balls. Press every dough ball slightly to make a hole in the center and put your ball on the baking mat.
4. Brush the top of every bagel with the remaining egg and top with sesame seeds.
5. Bake for about 15 minutes.

NUTRITION:

Calories: 469; Fat: 39g; Protein: 23g; Carbohydrates: 9g.

SATURDAY - DAY 6 - LUNCH
HEALTHY CELERY SOUP

Preparation Time: 10 minutes

Cooking Time: 20 minutes

Servings: 4

INGREDIENTS:

- 3 cups celery, chopped
- 1 cup vegetable broth
- 5 ounces cream cheese
- 1 ½ tablespoons fresh basil, chopped
- ¼ cup onion, chopped
- 1 tablespoon garlic, chopped
- 1 tablespoon olive oil
- ¼ teaspoon pepper
- ½ teaspoon salt

DIRECTIONS:

1. Heat some oil.
2. Add celery, onion and garlic to the saucepan and sauté for 4-5 minutes or until softened.
3. Add broth and bring to boil. Turn heat to low and simmer.
4. Add basil and cream cheese and stir until cheese is melted.
5. Season soup with pepper and salt.
6. Puree the soup until smooth.
7. Serve and enjoy.

NUTRITION:

Calories: 201; Fat: 5.4g; Protein: 5.1g; Carbohydrates: 3.9g.

SATURDAY - DAY 6 - DINNER
WINTER COMFORT STEW

Preparation Time: 15 minutes

Cooking Time: 50 minutes

Servings: 6

INGREDIENTS:

- 2 tablespoons olive oil
- 1 small yellow onion, chopped
- 2 garlic cloves, chopped
- 2 pounds grass-fed beef chuck, cut into 1-inch cubes
- 1 (14-ounce) can sugar-free crushed tomatoes
- 2 teaspoons ground allspice
- 1 ½ teaspoons red pepper flakes
- ½ cup homemade beef broth
- 6 ounces green olives, pitted
- 8 ounces fresh baby spinach
- 2 tablespoons fresh lemon juice
- Salt and freshly ground black pepper, to taste
- ¼ fresh cilantro, chopped

DIRECTIONS:

1. In a pan, heat the oil over high heat and sauté the onion and garlic for about 2-3 minutes.
2. Add the beef and cook for about 3-4 minutes or until browned, stirring frequently.
3. Add the tomatoes, spices and broth and bring to a boil.
4. Reduce the heat to low and simmer, covered for about 30-40 minutes or until the desired doneness of the beef.
5. Stir in the olives and spinach and simmer for about 2-3 minutes.
6. Stir in the lemon juice, salt, and black pepper and remove from the heat.
7. Serve hot with the garnishing of cilantro.

NUTRITION:

Calories: 388; Fat: 17.7g; Protein: 48.5g; Carbohydrates: 8g.

SUNDAY - DAY 7 - BREAKFAST
MATCHA GREEN JUICE

Preparation Time: 10 minutes

Cooking Time: 0 minutes

Servings: 2

INGREDIENTS:

- 5 ounces fresh kale
- 2 ounces fresh arugula
- ¼ cup fresh parsley
- 4 celery stalks
- 1 (1-inch) piece fresh ginger, peeled
- 1 lemon, peeled
- ½ teaspoon matcha green tea

DIRECTIONS:

1. Add all ingredients into a juicer and extract the juice according to the manufacturer's method.
2. Pour into 2 glasses and serve immediately.

NUTRITION:

Calories: 113; Fat: 2.1g; Protein: 1.3g; Carbohydrates: 12.3g.

SUNDAY - DAY 7 - LUNCH
LEMONY SALMON

Preparation Time: 10 minutes

Cooking Time: 10 minutes

Servings: 4

INGREDIENTS:

1 tablespoon butter, melted

1 tablespoon fresh lemon juice

1 teaspoon Worcestershire sauce

1 teaspoon lemon zest, grated finely.

4 (6-ounce) salmon fillets

Salt and ground black pepper, to taste

DIRECTIONS:

1. In a baking dish, place butter, lemon juice, Worcestershire sauce, and lemon zest, and mix well.
2. Coat the fillets with the mixture and then arrange skin side-up in the baking dish.
3. Set aside for about 15 minutes.
4. Preheat the broiler of the oven.
5. Arrange the oven rack about 6-inch from the heating element.
6. Line a broiler pan with a piece of foil.
7. Remove the salmon fillets from the baking dish and season with salt and black pepper.
8. Arrange the salmon fillets onto the prepared broiler pan, skin side down.
9. Broil for about 8-10 minutes.
10. Serve hot.

NUTRITION:

Calories: 253; Fat: 13.4g; Protein: 33.1g; Carbohydrates: 0.4g.

SUNDAY - DAY 7 - DINNER
YUMMY CHICKEN SKEWERS

Preparation Time: 10 minutes

Cooking Time: 10 minutes

Servings: 8

INGREDIENTS:

- 2 pounds chicken breast tenderloins
- 1 teaspoon lemon pepper seasoning
- 1 teaspoon garlic, minced
- 1 tablespoon olive oil
- 1 cup of salsa

DIRECTIONS:

1. Add chicken in a zip-lock bag along with 1/4 cup salsa, lemon pepper seasoning, garlic, and oil.
2. Seal bag and shake well and place it in the refrigerator overnight.
3. Thread marinated chicken onto the soaked wooden skewers.
4. Place skewers on hot grill and cooks for 8-10 minutes.
5. Brush with remaining salsa during the last 3 minutes of grilling.
6. Serve and enjoy.

NUTRITION:

Calories: 125; Fat: 2.5g; Protein: 24g; Carbohydrates: 2.1g.

WEEK 2

MONDAY - DAY 8 - BREAKFAST
COFFEE SURPRISE

Preparation Time: 5 minutes

Cooking Time: 5 minutes

Servings: 1 serving

INGREDIENTS:

2 heaped tablespoons flaxseed, ground

100ml cooking cream 35% Fat

½ teaspoon cocoa powder, dark and unsweetened

1 tablespoon goji berries

Freshly brewed coffee

DIRECTIONS:

1. Mix together the flaxseeds, cream and cocoa and coffee.
2. Season with goji berries.
3. Serve!

NUTRITION:

Calories: 55; Fat: 45g; Protein: 15g; Carbohydrates: 3g.

MONDAY - DAY 8 - LUNCH
BEEF SALAD WITH VEGETABLES

Preparation Time: 10 Minutes

Cooking Time: 10 Minutes

Servings: 4

INGREDIENTS:

1-pound (454 g) ground beef

¼ cup pork rinds, crushed

1 egg, whisked

1 onion, grated

1 tablespoon fresh parsley, chopped

½ teaspoon dried oregano

1 garlic clove, minced

Salt and black pepper, to taste

2 tablespoons olive oil, divided

Salad:

1 cup chopped arugula

1 cucumber, sliced

1 cup cherry tomatoes, halved

1 ½ tablespoons lemon juice

Salt and pepper, to taste

DIRECTIONS:

1. Stir together the beef, pork rinds, whisked egg, onion, parsley, oregano, garlic, salt, and pepper in a large bowl until completely mixed.
2. Make the meatballs: On a lightly floured surface, using a cookie scoop to scoop out equal-sized amounts of the beef mixture and form into meatballs with your palm.

3. Heat 1 tablespoon olive oil in a large skillet over medium heat, fry the meatballs for about 4 minutes on each side until cooked through.

4. Remove from the heat and set aside on a plate to cool.

5. In a salad bowl, mix the arugula, cucumber, cherry tomatoes, 1 tablespoon olive oil, and lemon juice. Serve, season with salt and pepper.

NUTRITION:

Calories: 302; Fat: 13g; Protein: 7g; Carbohydrates: 6g.

MONDAY - DAY 8 - DINNER
CRAB-STUFFED AVOCADO

Preparation Time: 20 minutes

Cooking Time: 0 minutes

Servings: 2

INGREDIENTS:

- 1 avocado, peeled, halved lengthwise, and pitted
- ½ teaspoon freshly squeezed lemon juice
- 4 ½ ounces Dungeness crabmeat
- ½ cup cream cheese
- ¼ cup chopped red bell pepper
- ¼ cup chopped, peeled English cucumber
- ½ scallion, chopped
- 1 teaspoon chopped cilantro
- Pinch sea salt
- Freshly ground black pepper

DIRECTIONS:

1. Brush the cut edges of the avocado with the lemon juice and set the halves aside on a plate.
2. In a bowl or container, the crabmeat, cream cheese, red pepper, cucumber, scallion, cilantro, salt, and pepper must be well-mixed.
3. Divide the crab mixture between the avocado.
4. Serve and enjoy.

NUTRITION:

Calories: 239; Fat: 11.4g; Protein: 5.9g; Carbohydrates: 3.8g.

TUESDAY - DAY 9 - BREAKFAST
COCONUT PILLOW

Preparation Time: 10 minutes

Cooking Time: 0 minutes

Servings: 4 servings

INGREDIENTS:

1 can unsweetened coconut milk

Berries of choice

Dark chocolate

DIRECTIONS:

1. Refrigerate the coconut milk for 24 hours.
2. Remove it from your refrigerator and whip for 2-3 minutes.
3. Fold in the berries.
4. Season with the chocolate shavings.
5. Serve!

NUTRITION:

Calories: 50; Fat: 5g; Protein: 1g; Carbohydrates: 2g.

TUESDAY - DAY 9 - LUNCH
PARMESAN CHICKEN

Preparation Time: 10 minutes

Cooking Time: 35 minutes

Servings: 4

INGREDIENTS:

- 1 pound chicken breasts, skinless and boneless
- ½ cup parmesan cheese, grated
- ¾ cup mayonnaise
- 1 teaspoon garlic powder
- ½ teaspoon Italian seasoning

DIRECTIONS:

1. Preheat the oven to 375°F.
2. Spray baking dish with cooking spray.
3. In a small bowl, mix together mayonnaise, garlic powder, poultry seasoning, and pepper.
4. Place chicken breasts into the prepared baking dish.
5. Spread mayonnaise mixture over chicken then sprinkles cheese on top of chicken.
6. Bake chicken for 35 minutes.
7. Serve and enjoy.

NUTRITION:

Calories: 391; Fat: 23g; Protein: 16g; Carbohydrates: 11g.

TUESDAY - DAY 9 - DINNER

DELICIOUS TOMATO BASIL SOUP

Preparation Time: 10 minutes

Cooking Time: 40 minutes

Servings: 4

INGREDIENTS:

¼ cup olive oil

½ cup heavy cream

1 pound tomatoes, fresh

4 cups chicken broth, divided

4 cloves garlic, fresh

Sea salt and pepper to taste

DIRECTIONS:

1. Preheat oven to 400°F and line a baking sheet with foil.
2. Remove the cores from your tomatoes and place them on the baking sheet along with the cloves of garlic.
3. Drizzle the tomatoes and garlic with olive oil, salt, and pepper.
4. Roast at 400°F for 30 minutes.
5. Pull the tomatoes out of the oven and place into a blender, along with the juices that have dripped onto the pan during roasting.
6. Add two cups of the chicken broth to the blender.
7. Blend until smooth, then strain the mixture into a large saucepan or a pot.
8. While the pan is on the stove, whisk the remaining two cups of broth and the cream into the soup.
9. Simmer for about ten minutes.
10. Season to taste, then serve hot!

NUTRITION:

Calories: 225; Fat: 20g; Protein: 6.5g; Carbohydrates: 5.5g.

WEDNESDAY - DAY 10 - BREAKFAST
ALMOND COCONUT EGG WRAPS

Preparation Time: 5 minutes

Cooking Time: 5 minutes

Servings: 4

INGREDIENTS:

- 5 organic eggs
- 1 tablespoon coconut flour
- 2 ½ teaspoons sea salt
- 2 tablespoons almond meal

DIRECTIONS:

1. Combine the ingredients in a blender and work them until creamy. Heat a skillet using the med-high temperature setting.

2. Pour two tablespoons of batter into the skillet and cook - covered for about three minutes. Turnover and cook for another 3 minutes. Serve the wraps piping hot.

NUTRITION:

Calories: 111; Fat: 8g; Protein: 8g; Carbohydrates: 3g.

WEDNESDAY - DAY 10 - LUNCH
CREAMED SPINACH

Preparation Time: 10 minutes

Cooking Time: 15 minutes

Servings: 4

INGREDIENTS:

- 2 tablespoons unsalted butter
- 1 small yellow onion, chopped
- 1 cup cream cheese, softened
- 2 (10-ounce) packages frozen spinach, thawed and squeezed dry
- 2-3 tablespoons water
- Salt and ground black pepper, as required
- 1 teaspoon fresh lemon juice

DIRECTIONS:

1. Melt some butter and sauté the onion for about 6–8 minutes.
2. Add the cream cheese and cook for about 2 minutes or until melted completely.
3. Stir in the water and spinach and cook for about 4–5 minutes.
4. Stir in the salt, black pepper, and lemon juice, and remove from heat.
5. Serve immediately.

NUTRITION:

Calories: 214; Fat: 9.5g; Protein: 4.2g; Carbohydrates: 2.1g.

WEDNESDAY - DAY 10 - DINNER
BEEF & MUSHROOM CHILI

Preparation Time: 15 minutes

Cooking Time: 3 hours 10 minutes

Servings: 8

INGREDIENTS:

- 2 pounds grass-fed ground beef
- 1 yellow onion
- ½ cup green bell pepper
- ½ cup carrot
- 4 ounces mushrooms
- 2 garlic cloves
- 1 can sugar-free tomato paste
- 2 tablespoons red chili powder
- 1 tablespoon ground cumin
- 1 teaspoon ground cinnamon
- 1 teaspoon red pepper flakes
- ½ teaspoon ground allspice
- Salt
- Ground black pepper
- 4 cups water
- ½ cup sour cream

DIRECTIONS:

1. Cook the beef for 8-10 minutes.
2. Stir in the remaining ingredient, except for the sour cream, and boil.
3. Cook on low, covered, for 3 hours.
4. Top with sour cream and serve.

NUTRITION:

Calories: 246; Fat: 15g; Protein: 25.1g; Carbohydrates: 8.2g.

THURSDAY - DAY 11 - BREAKFAST
BAGELS WITH CHEESE

Preparation Time: 10 minutes

Cooking Time: 15 minutes

Servings: 6

INGREDIENTS:

- 2 ½ cups Mozzarella cheese
- 1 teaspoon baking powder
- 3 ounces cream cheese
- 1 ½ cups almond flour
- 2 eggs

DIRECTIONS:

1. Shred the mozzarella and combine with the flour, baking powder, and cream cheese in a mixing container. Pop into the microwave for about one minute. Mix well.
2. Let the mixture cool and add the eggs. Break apart into six sections and shape into round bagels. Note: You can also sprinkle with a seasoning of your choice or pinch of salt if desired.
3. Bake them for approximately 12 to 15 minutes. Serve or cool and store.

NUTRITION:

Calories: 374; Fat: 31g; Protein: 19g; Carbohydrates: 8g.

THURSDAY - DAY 11 - LUNCH
PRAWNS SALAD WITH MIXED LETTUCE GREENS

Preparation Time: 10 Minutes

Cooking Time: 10 Minutes

Servings: 4

INGREDIENTS:

½ pound (227 g) prawns, peeled and deveined

Salt and chili pepper, to taste

1 tablespoon olive oil

2 cups mixed lettuce greens

For the dressing:

Mustard

Aioli

Lemon juice

DIRECTIONS:

1. In a bowl, add the prawns, salt, and chili pepper. Toss well.
2. Warm the olive oil over medium heat. Add the seasoned prawns and fry for about 6 to 8 minutes, stirring occasionally, or until the prawns are opaque.
3. Remove from the heat and set the prawns aside on a platter.
4. Make the dressing: In a small bowl, mix the mustard, aioli, and lemon juice until creamy and smooth.
5. Make the salad: In a separate bowl, add the mixed lettuce greens. Pour the dressing over the greens and toss to combine.
6. Divide the salad among four serving plates and serve it alongside the prawns.

NUTRITION:

Calories: 228; Fat: 17g; Protein: 5g; Carbohydrates: 3g.

THURSDAY - DAY 11 - DINNER
SPICED JALAPENO BITES WITH TOMATO

Preparation Time: 10 minutes

Cooking Time: 0 minutes

Servings: 4

INGREDIENTS:

- 1 cup turkey ham, chopped
- ¼ jalapeño pepper, minced
- ¼ cup mayonnaise
- 1/3 tablespoon Dijon mustard
- 4 tomatoes, sliced
- Salt and black pepper, to taste
- 1 tablespoon parsley, chopped

DIRECTIONS:

1. In a bowl, mix the turkey ham, jalapeño pepper, mayo, mustard, salt, and pepper.
2. Spread out the tomato slices on four serving plates, then top each plate with a spoonful of turkey ham mixture.
3. Serve garnished with chopped parsley.

NUTRITION:

Calories: 250; Fat: 14.1g; Protein: 18.9g; Carbohydrates: 4.1g.

FRIDAY - DAY 12 - BREAKFAST
BACON & EGG BREAKFAST MUFFINS

Preparation Time: 15 minutes

Cooking Time: 30 minutes

Servings: 12

INGREDIENTS:

- 8 large eggs
- 8 slices bacon
- 2 green onions

DIRECTIONS:

1. Warm the oven at 350°F. Spritz the muffin tin wells using a cooking oil spray. Chop the onions and set aside.

2. Prepare a large skillet using the medium temperature setting. Fry the bacon until it's crispy and place on a layer of paper towels to drain the grease. Chop it into small pieces after it has cooled.

3. Whisk the eggs, bacon, and green onions, mixing well until all of the ingredients are incorporated. Place the egg mixture into the muffin tin (halfway full). Bake it for about 20 to 25 minutes. Cool slightly and serve.

NUTRITION:

Calories: 117; Fat: 8.6g; Protein: 8.9g; Carbohydrates: 0.6g.

FRIDAY - DAY 12 – LUNCH
MEATLESS CABBAGE ROLLS

Preparation Time: 25 minutes

Cooking Time: 25 minutes,

Servings: 8,

INGREDIENTS:

For Filling:

1 ½ cups fresh button mushrooms, chopped

3 ¼ cups zucchini, chopped

1 cup red bell pepper, seeded and chopped

1 cup green bell pepper, seeded and chopped

½ teaspoon dried thyme, crushed

½ teaspoon dried marjoram, crushed

½ teaspoon dried basil, crushed

Salt and freshly ground black pepper, to taste

½ cup homemade vegetable broth

2 teaspoon fresh lemon juice

For Rolls:

8 large cabbage leaves, rinsed

8 ounces sugar-free tomato sauce

3 tablespoons fresh basil leaves, chopped

DIRECTIONS:

1. Preheat the oven to 400°F. Lightly, grease a 13x9-inch casserole dish.
2. For filling: in a large pan, add all the ingredients except the lemon juice over medium heat and bring to a boil.
3. Reduce the heat to low and simmer, covered for about 5 minutes.
4. Remove from the heat and set aside for about 5 minutes.

5. Add the lemon juice and stir to combine.
6. Meanwhile, for rolls: in a large pan of boiling water, add the cabbage leaves and boil for about 2-4 minutes.
7. Drain the cabbage leaves well.
8. Carefully, pat dry each cabbage leaf with paper towels.
9. Arrange the cabbage leaves onto a smooth surface.
10. With a knife, make a V shape cut in each leaf by cutting the thick vein.
11. Carefully, overlap the cut ends of each leaf.
12. Place the filling mixture over each leaf evenly and fold in the sides.
13. Then, roll each leaf to seal the filling and secure each with a toothpick.
14. In the bottom of the prepared casserole dish, place 1/3 cup of the tomato sauce evenly.
15. Arrange the cabbage rolls over sauce in a single layer and top with remaining sauce evenly.
16. Cover the casserole dish and bake for about 15 minutes.
17. Remove from the oven and set aside, uncovered for about 5 minutes.
18. Serve warm, garnishing with basil.

NUTRITION:

Calories: 33; Fat: 0.4g; Protein: 2.2g; Carbohydrates: 8.5g.

FRIDAY - DAY 12 - DINNER
SPINACH & CHICKEN MEATBALLS

Preparation Time: 10 minutes

Cooking Time: 30 Minutes

Servings: 10

INGREDIENTS:

- 1 ½ pounds ground chicken
- 8 ounces Parmigiano-Reggiano cheese, grated
- 1 teaspoon garlic, minced
- 1 tablespoon Italian seasoning mix
- 1 egg, whisked
- 8 ounces spinach, chopped
- ½ teaspoon mustard seeds
- Sea salt and ground black pepper, to taste
- ½ teaspoon paprika

DIRECTIONS:

1. Mix the ingredients until everything is well incorporated.
2. Now, shape the meat mixture into meatballs. Transfer your meatballs to a baking sheet and brush them with nonstick cooking oil.
3. Bake in the preheated oven at 350°F for about 25 minutes or until golden brown. Serve with cocktail sticks and enjoy!

NUTRITION:

Calories: 207; Fat: 12.3g; Protein: 19.5g; Carbohydrates: 4.6g.

SATURDAY - DAY 13 - BREAKFAST
KALE CHIPS

Preparation Time: 5 minutes

Cooking Time: 12 minutes

Servings: 2

INGREDIENTS:

- 1 bunch kale, removed from the stems
- 2 tablespoons extra virgin olive oil
- 1 tablespoon garlic salt

DIRECTIONS:

1. Preheat your oven to 350°F.
2. Coat the kale with olive oil.
3. Arrange on a baking sheet.
4. Bake for 12 minutes.
5. Sprinkle with garlic salt.

NUTRITION:

Calories: 100; Fat: 7g; Protein: 2.4g; Carbohydrates: 8.5g.

SATURDAY - DAY 13 - LUNCH
KETO TACO SALAD

Preparation Time: 5 Minutes

Cooking Time: 20 Minutes

Servings: 4

INGREDIENTS:

- 1 pound ground beef
- 3 tablespoons olive oil
- A dash of pepper
- 1 tablespoon onion powder
- 1 tablespoon cumin
- 1 tablespoon minced garlic clove
- 1 chopped tomato
- ½ cup sour cream
- ½ cup black olives
- ¼ cup cheddar cheese
- 2 tablespoons cilantro
- 1 chopped green pepper

DIRECTIONS:

1. With a taco salad, you will be able to enjoy everything that you love about tacos with a lot fewer carbohydrates! Whether you prepare this for taco Tuesday or a quick lunch, it is sure to be a crowd-pleaser!
2. Start this recipe by taking out your grilling pan and place it over a moderate temperature. As it warms up, you can add in the olive oil and let that sizzle. When you are set, add in the green pepper, spices, and ground beef. You can also use ground turkey in this recipe if that is more your style. Cook these ingredients together for ten minutes or so.
3. Next, place some mixed greens into a bowl and cover with the meat mixture you just created. If you would like some extra flavor, sprinkle some cheddar cheese over the top, along with some sour cream.

NUTRITION:

Calories: 138; Fat: 27g; Protein: 18g; Carbohydrates: 7g.

SATURDAY - DAY 13 - DINNER
ROASTED MACKEREL

Preparation Time: 10 minutes

Cooking Time: 20 minutes

Servings: 2

INGREDIENTS:

2 (7-ounce) mackerel fillets

1 tablespoon butter, melted

Salt and ground black pepper, to taste

DIRECTIONS:

1. Preheat the oven to 350°F.
2. Arrange a rack in the middle of the oven.
3. Lightly, grease a baking dish.
4. Brush the fish fillets with melted butter and then season with salt and black pepper.
5. Arrange the fish fillets into the prepared baking dish in a single layer.
6. Bake for about 20 minutes.
7. Serve hot.

NUTRITION:

Calories: 571; Fat: 41.1g; Protein: 47.4g; Carbohydrates: 7g.

SUNDAY - DAY 14 - BREAKFAST
HERBED COCONUT FLOUR BREAD

Preparation Time: 10 minutes

Cooking Time: 3 Minutes

Servings: 2

INGREDIENTS:

- 4 tablespoons coconut flour
- ½ teaspoon baking powder
- ½ teaspoon dried thyme
- 2 tablespoons whipping cream
- 2 eggs

Seasoning:

- ½ teaspoon oregano
- 2 tablespoons avocado oil

DIRECTIONS:

1. Take a medium bowl, place all the ingredients in it and then whisk until incorporated and smooth batter comes together.
2. Distribute the mixture evenly between two mugs and then microwave for a minute and 30 seconds until cooked.
3. When done, take out bread from the mugs, cut it into slices, and then serve.

NUTRITION:

Calories: 309; Fat: 26.1g; Protein: 9.3g; Carbohydrates: 5.3g.

SUNDAY - DAY 14 - LUNCH
MEXICAN PORK STEW

Preparation Time: 15 minutes

Cooking Time: 2 hours 10 minutes

Servings: 2

INGREDIENTS:

3 tablespoons unsalted butter

2 ½ pounds boneless pork ribs, cut into ¾-inch cubes

1 large yellow onion, chopped

4 garlic cloves, crushed

1 ½ cups homemade chicken broth

2 (10-ounce) cans sugar-free diced tomatoes

1 cup canned roasted poblano chiles

2 teaspoons dried oregano

1 teaspoon ground cumin

Salt, to taste

¼ cup fresh cilantro, chopped

2 tablespoons fresh lime juice

DIRECTIONS:

1. In a large pan, melt the butter over medium-high heat and cook the pork, onions, and garlic for about 5 minutes or until browned.
2. Add the broth and scrape up the browned bits.
3. Add the tomatoes, poblano chiles, oregano, cumin, and salt and bring to a boil.
4. Reduce the heat to medium-low and simmer, covered for about 2 hours.
5. Stir in the fresh cilantro and lime juice and remove from heat.
6. Serve hot.

NUTRITION:

Calories: 288; Fat: 10.1g; Protein: 39.6g; Carbohydrates: 8.8g.

SUNDAY - DAY 14 - DINNER

COLD GREEN BEANS AND AVOCADO SOUP

Preparation Time: 15 minutes

Cooking Time: 15 minutes

Servings: 4

INGREDIENTS:

1 tablespoon butter

2 tablespoon almond oil

1 garlic clove, minced

1 cup (227 g) green beans (fresh or frozen)

¼ avocado

1 cup heavy cream

½ cup grated cheddar cheese + extra for garnish

½ teaspoon coconut aminos

Salt to taste

DIRECTIONS:

1. Heat the butter and almond oil in a large skillet and sauté the garlic for 30 seconds.
2. Add the green beans and stir-fry for 10 minutes or until tender.
3. Add the mixture to a food processor and top with the avocado, heavy cream, cheddar cheese, coconut aminos, and salt.
4. Blend the ingredients until smooth.
5. Pour the soup into serving bowls, cover with plastic wraps and chill in the fridge for at least 2 hours.
6. Enjoy afterward with a garnish of grated white sharp cheddar cheese

NUTRITION:

Calories: 301; Fat: 3.1g; Protein: 3.1g; Carbohydrates: 2.8g.

WEEK 3

MONDAY - DAY 15 - BREAKFAST
BACON WRAPPED ASPARAGUS

Preparation Time: 10 minutes

Cooking Time: 20 minutes

Servings: 6

INGREDIENTS:

1 ½ pounds asparagus spears, sliced in half

6 slices bacon

2 tablespoons olive oil

Salt and pepper to taste

DIRECTIONS:

1. Preheat your oven to 400°F.
2. Wrap a handful of asparagus with bacon.
3. Secure with a toothpick.
4. Drizzle with the olive oil.
5. Season with salt and pepper.
6. Bake in the oven for 20 minutes or until bacon is crispy.

NUTRITION:

Calories: 166; Fat: 12.8g; Protein: 9.5g; Carbohydrates: 4.7g.

MONDAY - DAY 15 - LUNCH
CREAMY BROCCOLI AND LEEK SOUP

Preparation Time: 5 minutes

Cooking Time: 25 minutes

Servings: 4

INGREDIENTS:

10 ounces broccoli

1 leek

8 ounces cream cheese

3 ounces butter

3 cups water

1 garlic clove

½ cup fresh basil

Salt and pepper

DIRECTIONS:

1. Rinse the leek and chop both parts finely. Slice the broccoli thinly.
2. Place the veggies in a pot and cover with water and then season them. Boil the water until the broccoli softens.
3. Add the florets and garlic, while lowering the heat.
4. Add in the cheese, butter, pepper, and basil. Blend until desired consistency: if too thick, use water; if you want to make it thicker, use a little bit of heavy cream.

NUTRITION:

Calories: 451; Fat: 37g; Protein: 10g; Carbohydrates: 4g.

MONDAY - DAY 15 - DINNER
GARLIC BAKED BUTTER CHICKEN

Preparation Time: 10 minutes

Cooking Time: 40 minutes

Servings: 4

INGREDIENTS:

1 tablespoon rosemary leaves, fresh

3 chicken breasts, boneless, skinless (approximately 12 ounces); washed and cleaned

1 stick butter (½ cup)

½ cup Italian cheese, low Fat and shredded

6 garlic cloves, minced

Fresh ground pepper and salt to taste

DIRECTIONS:

1. Grease a large-sized baking dish lightly with a pat of butter, and preheat your oven to 375°F.
2. Season the chicken breasts with pepper and salt to taste; arrange them in the prepared baking dish, preferably in a single layer; set aside.
3. Now, over medium heat in a large skillet; heat the butter until melted, and then cook the garlic until lightly browned, for 4 to 5 minutes, stirring every now and then. Keep an eye on the garlic; don't burn it.
4. Add the rosemary; give everything a good stir; remove the skillet from heat.
5. Transfer the already prepared garlic butter over the meat.
6. Bake in the preheated oven for 30 minutes.
7. Sprinkle cheese on top and cook until the cheese is completely melted, for a couple of more minutes.
8. Remove from oven and let stand for a couple of minutes. Transfer the cooked meat to large serving plates. Serve and enjoy.

NUTRITION:

Calories: 375; Fat: 27g; Protein: 30g; Carbohydrates: 2.3g.

TUESDAY - DAY 16 - BREAKFAST
SHEET PAN EGGS WITH VEGGIES AND PARMESAN

Preparation Time: 5 minutes

Cooking Time: 15 minutes

Servings: 4

INGREDIENTS:

6 large eggs, whisked

Salt and pepper

1 small red pepper, diced

1 small yellow onion, chopped

½ cup diced mushrooms

½ cup diced zucchini

½ cup freshly grated parmesan cheese

DIRECTIONS:

1. Preheat the oven to 350°F and grease cooking spray on a rimmed baking sheet.
2. In a cup, whisk the eggs with salt and pepper until sparkling.
3. Add the peppers, onions, mushrooms, and courgettes until well mixed.
4. Pour the mixture into the baking sheet and scatter over a layer of evenness.
5. Sprinkle with parmesan, and bake until the egg is set for 13 to 16 minutes.
6. Let it cool down slightly, then cut to squares for serving.

NUTRITION:

Calories: 180; Fat: 10g; Protein: 14.5g; Carbohydrates: 5g.

TUESDAY - DAY 16 - LUNCH
STEAK WITH CHEESE SAUCE

Preparation Time: 15 minutes

Cooking Time: 17 minutes

Servings: 4

INGREDIENTS:

18 ounces grass-fed filet mignon

Salt

Ground black pepper

2 tablespoons butter

½ cup yellow onion

5 ¼ ounces blue cheese

1 cup heavy cream

1 garlic clove

Ground nutmeg

DIRECTIONS:

1. Cook onion for 5-8 minutes. Add the blue cheese, heavy cream, garlic, nutmeg, salt, and black pepper and stir.
2. Cook for about 3-5 minutes.
3. Put salt and black pepper in filet mignon steaks. Cook the steaks for 4 minutes per side.
4. Transfer and set aside. Top with cheese sauce, then serve.

NUTRITION:

Calories: 521; Fat: 22.1g; Protein: 44.7g; Carbohydrates: 3.3g.

TUESDAY - DAY 16 - DINNER
SCRUMPTIOUS CAULIFLOWER CASSEROLE

Preparation Time: 15 minutes

Cooking Time: 40 minutes

Servings: 4

INGREDIENTS:

1 large head cauliflower, cut into florets

2 tablespoons butter

2 ounces cream cheese, softened

1 ¼ cups sharp cheddar cheese, shredded and divided

1 cup heavy cream

Salt and freshly ground black pepper, to taste

¼ cup scallion, chopped and divided

DIRECTIONS:

1. Preheat the oven to 350°F.
2. In a large pan of boiling water, add the cauliflower florets and cook for about 2 minutes.
3. Drain cauliflower and keep aside.
4. For the cheese sauce: in a medium pan, add butter over medium-low heat and cook until just melted.
5. Add cream cheese, 1 cup cheddar cheese, heavy cream, salt and black pepper and cook until melted and smooth, stirring continuously.
6. Remove from heat and keep aside to cool slightly.
7. In a baking dish, place cauliflower florets, cheese sauce, and 3 tablespoons of scallion and stir to combine well.
8. Sprinkle with remaining cheddar cheese and scallion.
9. Bake for about 30 minutes.
10. Remove the casserole dish from oven and set aside for about 5-10 minutes before serving.
11. Cut into 4 equal-sized portions and serve.

NUTRITION:

Calories: 365; Fat: 33.6g; Protein: 12g; Carbohydrates: 5.6g.

WEDNESDAY - DAY 17 - BREAKFAST
CRISPY CHAI WAFFLES

Preparation Time: 10 minutes

Cooking Time: 20 minutes

Servings: 4

INGREDIENTS:

4 large eggs, separated into whites and yolks

3 tablespoons coconut flour

3 tablespoons powdered erythritol

1 ¼ teaspoon baking powder

1 teaspoon vanilla extract

½ teaspoon ground cinnamon

¼ teaspoon ground ginger

Pinch ground cloves

Pinch ground cardamom

3 tablespoons coconut oil, melted

3 tablespoons unsweetened almond milk

Cocoa

DIRECTIONS:

1. Divide the eggs into two separate mixing bowls.
2. Whip the whites of the eggs until stiff peaks develop and then set aside.
3. Whisk the egg yolks into the other bowl with the coconut flour, erythritol, baking powder, cocoa, cinnamon, cardamom, and cloves.
4. Pour the melted coconut oil and the almond milk into the second bowl and whisk.
5. Fold softly in the whites of the egg until you have just combined.
6. Preheat waffle iron with cooking spray and grease.
7. Spoon into the iron for about 1/2 cup of batter.
8. Cook the waffle according to directions from the maker.
9. Move the waffle to a plate and repeat with the batter left over.

NUTRITION:

Calories: 215; Fat: 17g; Protein: 8g; Carbohydrates: 8g.

WEDNESDAY - DAY 17 - LUNCH
CREAMY KALE SALAD

Preparation Time: 15 minutes

Cooking Time: 0 minutes

Servings: 3

INGREDIENTS:

1 bunch spinach

1 ½ tablespoons lemon juice

1 cup sour cream

1 cup roasted macadamia

2 tablespoons sesame seeds oil

1 ½ garlic clove, minced

½ teaspoon black pepper

¼ teaspoon salt

2 tablespoons lime juice

1 bunch kale

Toppings

1 ½ avocado, diced

¼ cup pecans, chopped

DIRECTIONS:

1. Confirm that you have all the ingredients. Chop the kale, wash it, then remove the ribs.
2. Now transfer kale to a large bowl.
3. Add sour cream, lime juice, macadamia, sesame seeds oil, pepper, salt, garlic.
4. Finally, mix thoroughly. Top with your avocado and pecans. Serve and enjoy.

NUTRITION:

Calories: 291; Fat: 5.1g; Protein: 11.8g; Carbohydrates: 4.3g.

WEDNESDAY - DAY 17 - DINNER
SHRIMP CASSEROLE

Preparation Time: 15 minutes

Cooking Time: 30 minutes

Servings: 6

INGREDIENTS:

¼ cup unsalted butter

1 tablespoon garlic, minced

1 ½ pounds large shrimp, peeled and deveined

¾ teaspoon dried oregano, crushed

¼ teaspoon red pepper flakes, crushed

¼ cup fresh parsley, chopped

½ cup homemade chicken broth

1 tablespoon fresh lemon juice

1 (14½-ounce) can sugar-free diced tomatoes, drained

4 ounces feta cheese, crumbled

DIRECTIONS:

1. Preheat the oven to 350°F.
2. In a large wok, melt butter over medium-high heat and sauté the garlic for about 1 minute.
3. Add the shrimp, oregano and red pepper flakes and cook for about 4–5 minutes.
4. Stir in the parsley and salt and immediately transfer into a casserole dish evenly.
5. In the same wok, add broth and lemon juice over medium heat and simmer for about 2–3 minutes or until liquid reduces to half.
6. Stir in tomatoes and cook for about 2–3 minutes.
7. Pour the tomato mixture over shrimp mixture evenly and sprinkle with cheese.
8. Bake for approximately 15–20 minutes or until top becomes golden-brown.
9. Remove from the oven and serve hot.

NUTRITION:

Calories: 272; Fat: 13.9g; Protein: 29.8g; Carbohydrates: 6g.

THURSDAY - DAY 18 - BREAKFAST
BACON & AVOCADO OMELET

Preparation Time: 5 minutes

Cooking Time: 5 minutes

Servings: 1

INGREDIENTS:

- 1 slice crispy bacon
- 2 large organic eggs
- 5 cups freshly grated parmesan cheese
- 1 teaspoon finely chopped herbs
- 2 tablespoons ghee or coconut oil or butter
- Half 1 small avocado

DIRECTIONS:

1. Prepare the bacon to your liking and set aside. Combine the eggs, parmesan cheese, and your choice of finely chopped herbs. Warm a skillet and add the butter/ghee to melt using the medium-high heat setting. When the pan is hot, whisk and add the eggs.
2. Prepare the omelet, working it towards the middle of the pan for about 30 seconds. When firm, flip and cook it for another 30 seconds. Arrange the omelet on a plate and garnish with the crunched bacon bits. Serve with sliced avocado.

NUTRITION:

Calories: 719; Fat: 63g; Protein: 30g; Carbohydrates: 3.3g.

THURSDAY - DAY 18 - LUNCH
VEGETABLE PATTIES

Preparation Time: 15 minutes

Cooking Time: 35 minutes

Servings: 4

INGREDIENTS:

- 1 tablespoon olive oil
- 1 onion, chopped
- 1 garlic clove, minced
- 1/2 head cauliflower, grated
- 1 carrot, shredded
- 3 tablespoons coconut flour
- 1/2 cup Gruyere cheese, shredded
- 1/2 cup Parmesan cheese, grated
- 2 eggs, beaten
- 1/2 teaspoon dried rosemary
- Salt and black pepper, to taste

DIRECTIONS:

1. Cook onion and garlic in warm olive oil over medium heat, until soft, for about 3 minutes.
2. Stir in grated cauliflower and carrot and cook for a minute; allow cooling and set aside.
3. To the cooled vegetables, add the rest of the ingredients, form balls from the mixture, then press each ball to form a burger patty.
4. Set oven to 400°F and bake the burgers for 20 minutes.
5. Flip and bake for another 10 minutes or until the top becomes golden brown.

NUTRITION:

Calories: 315; Fat: 12.1g; Protein: 5.8g; Carbohydrates: 3.3g.

THURSDAY - DAY 18 - DINNER
CHICKEN ENCHILADA SOUP

Preparation Time: 10 minutes

Cooking Time: 45 minutes

Servings: 4

INGREDIENTS:

½ cup fresh cilantro, chopped

1 ¼ teaspoons chili powder

1 cup fresh tomatoes, diced

1 medium yellow onion, diced

1 small red bell pepper, diced

1 tablespoon cumin, ground

1 tablespoon extra-virgin olive oil

1 tablespoon lime juice, fresh

1 teaspoon dried oregano

2 cloves garlic, minced

2 large stalks celery, diced

4 cups chicken broth

8 ounces chicken thighs, boneless & skinless, shredded

8 ounces cream cheese, softened

DIRECTIONS:

1. In a pot over medium heat, warm olive oil.
2. Once hot, add celery, red pepper, onion, and garlic. Cook for about 3 minutes or until shiny.
3. Stir the tomatoes into the pot and let cook for another 2 minutes.
4. Add seasonings to the pot, stir in chicken broth and bring to a boil.
5. Once boiling, drop the heat to low and allow to simmer for 20 minutes.

6. Once simmered, add the cream cheese and allow the soup to return to a boil.
7. Drop the heat once again and let it simmer for another 20 minutes.
8. Stir the shredded chicken into the soup, along with the lime juice and the cilantro.
9. Spoon into bowls and serve hot!

NUTRITION:

Calories: 420; Fat: 29.5g; Protein: 27g; Carbohydrates: 12g.

FRIDAY - DAY 19 - BREAKFAST
CLASSIC WESTERN OMELET

Preparation Time: 5 minutes

Cooking Time: 10 minutes

Servings: 1

INGREDIENTS:

- 2 teaspoons coconut oil
- 3 large eggs, whisked
- 1 tablespoon heavy cream
- Salt and pepper
- ¼ cup diced green pepper
- ¼ cup diced yellow onion
- ¼ cup diced ham

DIRECTIONS:

1. In a small bowl, whisk the eggs, heavy cream, salt, and pepper.
2. Heat up 1 teaspoon of coconut oil over medium heat in a small skillet.
3. Add the peppers and onions, then sauté the ham for 3 to 4 minutes.
4. Spoon the mixture in a cup, and heat the skillet with the remaining oil.
5. Pour in the whisked eggs and cook until the egg's bottom begins to set.
6. Tilt the pan and cook until almost set to spread the egg.
7. Spoon the ham and veggie mixture over half of the omelet and turn over.
8. Let cook the omelet until the eggs are set and then serve hot.

NUTRITION:

Calories: 415; Fat: 32.5g; Protein: 2.5g; Carbohydrates: 6.5g.

FRIDAY - DAY 19 - LUNCH
HERBED SALMON

Preparation Time: 10 minutes

Cooking Time: 8 minutes

Servings: 4

INGREDIENTS:

- 2 garlic cloves, minced
- 1 teaspoon dried oregano, crushed
- 1 teaspoon dried basil, crushed
- Salt and ground black pepper, to taste
- ¼ cup olive oil
- 2 tablespoons fresh lemon juice
- 4 (4-ounce) salmon fillets

DIRECTIONS:

1. For salmon: In a large bowl, add all ingredients (except salmon) and mix well.
2. Add salmon and coat with marinade generously.
3. Cover and refrigerate to marinate for at least 1 hour.
4. Preheat the grill to medium-high heat. Grease the grill grate.
5. Place the salmon onto the grill and cook for about 4 minutes per side.
6. Serve hot.

NUTRITION:

Calories: 263; Fat: 19.7g; Protein: 22.2g; Carbohydrates: 0.9g.

FRIDAY - DAY 19 - DINNER
SPINACH AND ZUCCHINI LASAGNA

Preparation Time: 15 minutes

Cooking Time: 45 minutes

Servings: 4

INGREDIENTS:

2 zucchinis, sliced

Salt and black pepper to taste

2 cups ricotta cheese

2 cups shredded mozzarella cheese

3 cups tomato sauce

1 cup baby spinach

DIRECTIONS:

1. Let the oven heat to 375° and grease a baking dish with cooking spray.
2. Put the zucchini slices in a colander and sprinkle with salt.
3. Let sit and drain liquid for 5 minutes and pat dry with paper towels.
4. Mix the ricotta, mozzarella cheese, salt, and black pepper to evenly combine and spread 1/4 cup of the mixture in the bottom of the baking dish.
5. Layer 1/3 of the zucchini slices on top spread 1 cup of tomato sauce over, and scatter a 1/3 cup of spinach on top. Repeat process.
6. Grease one end of foil with cooking spray and cover the baking dish with the foil.
7. Let it bake for about 35 minutes. And bake further for 5 to 10 minutes or until the cheese has a nice golden-brown color.
8. Remove the dish, sit for 5 minutes, make slices of the lasagna, and serve warm.

NUTRITION:

Calories: 376; Fat: 14.1g; Protein: 9.5g; Carbohydrates: 2.1g.

SATURDAY - DAY 20 - BREAKFAST
FIVE GREENS SMOOTHIE

Preparation Time: 10 minutes

Cooking Time: 0 minutes

Servings: 3

INGREDIENTS:

- 6 kale leaves, chopped
- 3 celery stalks, chopped
- 1 ripe avocado, skinned, pitted, sliced
- 1 cup of ice cubes
- 2 cups spinach, chopped
- 1 large cucumber, peeled and chopped
- Chia seeds to garnish

DIRECTIONS:

1. In a blender, add the kale, celery, avocado, and ice cubes, and blend for 45 seconds. Add the spinach and cucumber, and process for another 45 seconds until smooth.
2. Pour the smoothie into glasses, garnish with chia seeds, and serve the drink immediately.

NUTRITION:

Calories: 124; Fat: 7.8g; Protein: 3.2g; Carbohydrates: 3.5g.

SATURDAY - DAY 20 - LUNCH
OMELET-STUFFED PEPPERS

Preparation Time: 5 minutes

Cooking Time: 20 minutes

Servings: 2

INGREDIENTS

1 large green bell pepper, halved, cored

2 eggs

2 slices of bacon, chopped, cooked

2 tablespoons grated parmesan cheese

Seasoning:

1/3 teaspoon salt

¼ teaspoon ground black pepper

DIRECTIONS:

1. Turn on the oven, then set it to 400°F, and let preheat.
2. Then take a baking dish, pour in 1 tbsp. water, place bell pepper halved in it, cut-side up, and bake for 5 minutes.
3. Meanwhile, crack eggs in a bowl, add chopped bacon and cheese, season with salt and black pepper, and whisk until combined.
4. After 5 minutes of baking time, remove the baking dish from the oven, evenly fill the peppers with egg mixture and continue baking for 15 to 20 minutes until eggs have set.
5. Serve.

NUTRITION:

Calories: 428; Fat: 35.2g; Protein: 23.5g; Carbohydrates: 4.3g.

SATURDAY - DAY 20 - DINNER
WEEKEND DINNER STEW

Preparation Time: 15 minutes

Cooking Time: 55 minutes

Servings: 6

INGREDIENTS:

- 1 ½ pounds grass-fed beef stew meat, trimmed and cubed into 1-inch size
- Salt and freshly ground black pepper, to taste
- 1 tablespoon olive oil
- 1 cup homemade tomato puree
- 4 cups homemade beef broth
- 2 cups zucchini, chopped
- 2 celery ribs, sliced
- ½ cup carrots, peeled and sliced
- 2 garlic cloves, minced
- ½ tablespoon dried thyme
- 1 teaspoon dried parsley
- 1 teaspoon dried rosemary
- 1 tablespoon paprika
- 1 teaspoon onion powder
- 1 teaspoon garlic powder

DIRECTIONS:

1. In a large bowl, add the beef cubes, salt, and black pepper and toss to coat well.
2. In a large pan, heat the oil over medium-high heat and cook the beef cubes for about 4-5 minutes or until browned.
3. Add the remaining ingredients and stir to combine.
4. Increase the heat to high and bring to a boil.

5. Reduce the heat to low and simmer, covered for about 40-50 minutes.
6. Stir in the salt and black pepper and remove from the heat.
7. Serve hot.

NUTRITION:

Calories: 293; Fat: 10.7g; Protein: 9.3g; Carbohydrates: 8g.

SUNDAY - DAY 21 - BREAKFAST
BACON & CHEESE FRITTATA

Preparation Time: 5 minutes

Cooking Time: 35 minutes

Servings: 6

INGREDIENTS:

- 1 cup heavy cream
- 6 eggs
- 5 crispy slices of bacon
- 2 chopped green onions
- 4 ounces cheddar cheese

DIRECTIONS:

1. Warm the oven temperature to reach 350°F.
2. Whisk the eggs and seasonings. Empty into the pie pan and top off with the remainder of the ingredients. Bake for 30-35 minutes. Wait for a few minutes before serving for best results.

NUTRITION:

Calories: 320; Fat: 29g; Protein: 13g; Carbohydrates: 2g.

SUNDAY - DAY 21 - LUNCH
LEMON ROSEMARY CHICKEN THIGHS

Preparation Time: 10 minutes

Cooking Time: 45 minutes

Servings: 4

INGREDIENTS:

4 chicken thighs, skinless

2 garlic cloves, roughly chopped

4 sprigs of Rosemary, fresh

1 lemon, medium

2 tablespoons butter

Pepper, and salt to taste

DIRECTIONS:

1. Preheat your oven to 400°F in advance and heat up a cast-iron skillet over high heat as well.
2. Season both sides of the meat with pepper, and salt. When the skillet is hot; carefully place the coated thighs, preferably skin side down into the hot skillet, and sear them for 4 to 5 minutes, until nicely brown.
3. Carefully flip and flavor the thighs with the lemon juice (only use ½ of the lemon). Quarter the leftover lemon halves and throw the pieces into the pan with the chicken.
4. Add the chopped garlic cloves together with some rosemary into the skillet.
5. Place the skillet inside the oven and bake for 30 minutes.
6. Remove the skillet from the oven. To add flavor, moisture, and more crispiness; add a portion of butter over the chicken thighs. Bake for 10 more minutes.
7. Serve hot and enjoy.

NUTRITION:

Calories: 159; Fat: 8.8g; Protein: 13.9g; Carbohydrates: 6.9g.

SUNDAY - DAY 21 - DINNER
NEW ENGLAND SALMON PIE

Preparation Time: 20 minutes

Cooking Time: 50 minutes

Servings: 5

INGREDIENTS:

For Crust:

¾ cup almond flour

4 tablespoons coconut flour

4 tablespoons sesame seeds

1 tablespoon psyllium husk powder

1 teaspoon organic baking powder

Pinch of salt

1 organic egg

3 tablespoons olive oil

4 tablespoons water

For Filling:

8 ounces salmon fillets

4 ¼ ounces cream cheese, softened

1 ¼ cups cheddar cheese, shredded

1 cup mayonnaise

3 organic eggs

2 tablespoons fresh dill, finely chopped

½ teaspoon onion powder

¼ teaspoon ground black pepper

DIRECTIONS:

1. Preheat the oven to 350°F. Line a 10-inch springform pan with parchment paper.
2. For crust: place all the ingredients in a food processor, fitted with a plastic pastry blade and pulse until a dough ball is formed.
3. Place the dough into prepared springform pan and with your fingers, gently press in the bottom.
4. Bake for about 12-15 minutes or until lightly browned.
5. Remove the pie crust from the oven and let it cool slightly.
6. Meanwhile, for filling: in a bowl add all the ingredients and mix well.
7. Place the cheese mixture over the pie crust evenly.
8. Bake for about 35 minutes or until the pie is golden brown.
9. Remove the pie from oven and let it cool slightly.
10. Cut into 5 equal-sized slices and serve warm.

NUTRITION:

Calories: 762; Fat: 70g; Protein: 24.8g; Carbohydrates: 10.8g.

WEEK 4

MONDAY - DAY 22 - BREAKFAST
ITALIAN-STYLE ASPARAGUS WITH CHEESE

Preparation Time: 10 minutes

Cooking Time: 10 Minutes

Servings: 2

INGREDIENTS:

- ½ pound asparagus spears, trimmed, cut into bite-sized pieces
- 1 teaspoon Italian spice blend
- ½ tablespoon lemon juice
- 1 tablespoon extra-virgin olive oil
- 4 tablespoons Romano cheese, freshly grated

DIRECTIONS:

1. Bring a saucepan of lightly salted water to a boil. Turn the heat to medium-low. Add the asparagus spears and cook for approximately 3 minutes. Drain and transfer to a serving bowl.
2. Add the Italian spice blend, lemon juice, and extra-virgin olive oil; toss until well coated.
3. Top with Romano cheese and serve immediately. Bon appétit!

NUTRITION:

Calories: 193; Fat: 14.1g; Protein: 11.5g; Carbohydrates: 5.6g.

MONDAY - DAY 22 - LUNCH
FRESH SUMMER SALAD

Preparation Time: 3 Minutes

Cooking Time: 0 Minutes

Servings: 4

INGREDIENTS:

- 2 tablespoons olive oil
- 1 tablespoon thyme
- 1 tablespoon oregano
- ¼ cup ricotta cheese
- 1 leaf, chopped basil
- 1 tablespoon balsamic vinegar
- 1 sliced cucumber
- 3 sliced tomatoes
- 5 sliced radishes
- 1 sliced onion

DIRECTIONS:

Don't be fooled by the name; this salad can be enjoyed at any time of the year! If you are looking for a meatless dish, this is the perfect recipe for you!

1. The first step for this recipe is to make your ricotta cheese. You can complete this in a small bowl by mixing the thyme, oregano, basil with the ricotta cheese.

2. Next, make your own dressing! For this task, whisk your vinegar and olive oil together. Once this is complete, season however you like.

3. Finally, take some time to slice and dice the vegetables according to the directions above. When your veggies are all set, assemble them in your serving dishes and pour the dressing generously over the top. As a final touch, dollop your ricotta cheese over your salad, and then your salad will be ready for serving.

NUTRITION:

Calories: 158; Fat: 19g; Protein: 16g; Carbohydrates: 4g.

MONDAY - DAY 22 - DINNER
MEATBALLS CURRY

Preparation Time: 15 minutes

Cooking Time: 25 minutes

Servings: 6

INGREDIENTS:

For Meatballs:

1 pound lean ground pork

2 organic eggs

3 tablespoons yellow onion

¼ cup fresh parsley leaves

¼ teaspoon fresh ginger

2 garlic cloves

1 jalapeño pepper

1 teaspoon Erythritol

1 tablespoon red curry paste

3 tablespoons olive oil

For Curry:

1 yellow onion

Salt

2 garlic cloves

¼ teaspoon ginger

2 tablespoons red curry paste

1 can unsweetened coconut milk

Ground black pepper

¼ cup fresh parsley

DIRECTIONS:

For meatballs:

1. Mix all the ingredients for the meatballs, except oil. Make small-sized balls from the mixture.

2. Cook meatballs for 3-5 minutes. Transfer and put aside.

For curry:

3. Sauté onion and salt for 4-5 minutes. Add the garlic and ginger. Add the curry paste and sauté for 1-2 minutes. Add coconut milk, and meatballs, then simmer.

4. Simmer again for 10-12 minutes. Put salt and black pepper. Remove, then serve with fresh parsley.

NUTRITION:

Calories: 444; Fat: g; Protein: 17g; Carbohydrates: 8.6g.

TUESDAY - DAY 23 - BREAKFAST
BLT PARTY BITES

Preparation Time: 35 minutes

Cooking Time: 0 minute

Servings: 8

INGREDIENTS:

4 ounces bacon, chopped

3 tablespoons panko breadcrumbs

1 tablespoon Parmesan cheese, grated

1 teaspoon mayonnaise

1 teaspoon lemon juice

Salt to taste

½ heart Romaine lettuce, shredded

6 cocktail tomatoes

DIRECTIONS:

1. Put the bacon in a pan over medium heat.
2. Fry until crispy.
3. Transfer bacon to a plate lined with paper towel.
4. Add breadcrumbs and cook until crunchy.
5. Transfer breadcrumbs to another plate also lined with paper towel.
6. Sprinkle Parmesan cheese on top of the breadcrumbs.
7. Mix the mayonnaise, salt and lemon juice.
8. Toss the Romaine in the mayo mixture.
9. Slice each tomato on the bottom to create a flat surface so it can stand by itself.
10. Slice the top off as well.
11. Scoop out the insides of the tomatoes.
12. Stuff each tomato with the bacon, Parmesan, breadcrumbs and top with the lettuce.

NUTRITION:

Calories: 107; Fat: 6.5g; Protein: 6.5g; Carbohydrates: 5.4g.

TUESDAY - DAY 23 - LUNCH
GRILLED HALLOUMI CHEESE WITH EGGS

Preparation Time: 15 minutes

Cooking Time: 15 minutes

Servings: 4

INGREDIENTS:

- 4 slices Halloumi cheese
- 3 teaspoons olive oil
- 1 teaspoon dried Greek seasoning blend
- 1 tablespoon olive oil
- 6 eggs, beaten
- ½ teaspoon sea salt
- ¼ teaspoon crushed red pepper flakes
- 1 ½ cups avocado, pitted and sliced
- 1 cup grape tomatoes, halved
- 4 tablespoons pecans, chopped

DIRECTIONS:

1. Preheat your grill to medium.
2. Set the Halloumi in the center of a piece of heavy-duty foil.
3. Sprinkle oil over the Halloumi and apply the Greek seasoning blend.
4. Close the foil to create a packet.
5. Grill for about 15 minutes, then slice into four pieces.
6. In a frying pan, warm one tablespoon of oil and cook the eggs.
7. Stir well to create large and soft curds—season with salt and pepper.
8. Put the eggs and grilled cheese on a serving bowl.
9. Serve alongside tomatoes and avocado, decorated with chopped pecans.

NUTRITION:

Calories: 219; Fat: 5.1g; Protein: 3.9g; Carbohydrates: 1.5g.

TUESDAY - DAY 23 - DINNER
YELLOW CHICKEN SOUP

Preparation Time: 15 minutes

Cooking Time: 25 minutes

Servings: 5

INGREDIENTS:

2 ½ teaspoons ground turmeric

1 ½ teaspoons ground cumin

1/8 teaspoon cayenne pepper

2 tablespoons butter, divided

1 small yellow onion, chopped

2 cups cauliflower, chopped

2 cups broccoli, chopped

4 cups homemade chicken broth

1 ½ cups water

1 teaspoon fresh ginger root, grated

1 bay leaf

2 cups Swiss chard, stemmed and chopped finely

½ cup unsweetened coconut milk

3 (4-ounce) grass-fed boneless, skinless chicken thighs, cut into bite-size pieces

2 tablespoons fresh lime juice

DIRECTIONS:

1. In a small bowl, mix together the turmeric, cumin, and cayenne pepper and set aside.
2. In a large pan, melt 1 tablespoon of butter over medium heat and sauté the onion for about 3-4 minutes.
3. Add the cauliflower, broccoli, and half of the spice mixture and cook for another 3-4 minutes.

4. Add the broth, water, ginger, and bay leaf and bring to a boil.

5. Reduce the heat to low and simmer for about 8-10 minutes.

6. Stir in the Swiss chard and coconut milk and cook for about 1-2 minutes.

7. Meanwhile, in a large skillet, melt the remaining butter over medium heat and sear the chicken pieces for about 5 minutes.

8. Stir in the remaining spice mix and cook for about 5 minutes, stirring frequently.

9. Transfer the soup into serving bowls and top with the chicken pieces.

10. Drizzle with lime juice and serve.

NUTRITION:

Calories: 258; Fat: 16.8g; Protein: 18.4g; Carbohydrates: 8.4g.

WEDNESDAY - DAY 24 - BREAKFAST
ALMOND BUTTER MUFFINS

Preparation Time: 10 minutes

Cooking Time: 25 minutes

Servings: 6

INGREDIENTS:

- 1 cups almond flour
- ½ cup powdered erythritol
- 1 teaspoons baking powder
- ¼ teaspoon salt
- ¾ cup almond butter, warmed
- ¾ cup unsweetened almond milk
- 2 large eggs

DIRECTIONS:

1. Preheat the oven to 350°F, and line a paper liner muffin pan.
2. In a mixing bowl, whisk the almond flour and the erythritol, baking powder, and salt.
3. Whisk the almond milk, almond butter, and the eggs together in a separate bowl.
4. Drop the wet ingredients into the dry until just mixed together.
5. Spoon the batter into the prepared pan and bake for 22 to 25 minutes until clean comes out the knife inserted in the middle.
6. Let cool and enjoy.

NUTRITION:

Calories: 135; Fat: 11g; Protein: 6g; Carbohydrates: 4g.

WEDNESDAY - DAY 24 - LUNCH
GRILLED STEAK

Preparation Time: 15 minutes

Cooking Time: 12 minutes

Servings: 6

INGREDIENTS:

- 1 teaspoon lemon zest
- 1 garlic clove
- 1 tablespoon red chili powder
- 1 tablespoon paprika
- 1 tablespoon ground coffee
- Salt
- Ground black pepper
- 2 grass-fed skirt steaks

DIRECTIONS:

1. Mix all the ingredients except steaks. Marinate the steaks and keep aside for 30-40 minutes.
2. Grill the steaks for 5-6 minutes per side. Remove, then cool before slicing. Serve.

NUTRITION:

Calories: 473; Fat: 17.6g; Protein: 60.8g; Carbohydrates: 1.6g.

WEDNESDAY - DAY 24 - DINNER
TURKISH STYLE BELL PEPPERS

Preparation Time: 15 minutes

Cooking Time: 50 minutes

Servings: 4

INGREDIENTS:

- 4 large organic eggs
- ½ cup plus 2 tablespoons Parmesan cheese, grated and divided
- ½ cup mozzarella cheese, shredded
- ½ cup ricotta cheese
- 1 teaspoon garlic powder
- ¼ teaspoon dried parsley
- 2 medium bell peppers, cut in half and seeded
- ¼ cup fresh baby spinach leaves

DIRECTIONS:

1. Preheat the oven to 375°F and lightly, grease a baking dish.
2. In a small food processor, place the eggs, ½ cup of Parmesan, mozzarella, ricotta cheese, garlic powder and parsley and pulse until well combined.
3. Arrange the bell pepper halves into prepared baking dish, cut side up.
4. Place the cheese mixture into each pepper half and top each with a few spinach leaves.
5. With a fork, push the spinach leaves into the cheese mixture.
6. With a piece of foil, cover the baking dish and bake for about 35-45 minutes.
7. Now, set the oven to broiler on high.
8. Top each bell pepper half with the remaining Parmesan cheese and broil for about 3-5 minutes.
9. Remove from the oven and serve hot.

NUTRITION:

Calories: 191; Fat: 11.2g; Protein: 16.6g; Carbohydrates: 7g.

THURSDAY - DAY 25 - BREAKFAST
BERRY SOY YOGURT PARFAIT

Preparation Time: 2-4 minutes

Cooking Time: 0 minutes

Servings: 1

INGREDIENTS:

One carton vanilla cultured soy yogurt

¼ cup granola (gluten-free)

1 cup berries (you can take strawberries, blueberries, raspberries, blackberries)

DIRECTIONS:

1. Put half of the yogurt in a glass jar or serving dish.
2. On the top put half of the berries.
3. Then sprinkle with half of granola
4. Repeat layers.

NUTRITION:

Calories: 244; Fat: 3.1g; Protein: 1.4g; Carbohydrates: 11.3g.

THURSDAY - DAY 25 - LUNCH
SESAME CHICKEN SALAD

Preparation Time: 20 minutes

Cooking Time: 0 minutes

Servings: 4

INGREDIENTS:

1 tablespoon sesame seeds

1 cucumber, peeled, halved lengthwise, and sliced.

3.5 ounces cabbage, chopped

2 ounces pak choi, finely chopped

½ red onion, thinly sliced

0.7-ounce large parsley, chopped

5 ounces cooked chicken, minced

For the dressing:

1 tablespoon extra virgin olive oil

1 teaspoon sesame oil

1 lime juice

1 teaspoon light honey

2 teaspoons soy sauce

DIRECTIONS:

1. Roast your sesame seeds in a dry pan for 2 minutes until they become slightly golden and fragrant.
2. Transfer to a plate to cool.
3. In a small bowl, mix olive oil, sesame oil, lime juice, honey, and soy sauce to prepare the dressing.
4. Place the cucumber, black cabbage, pak-choi, red onion, and parsley in a large bowl and mix gently.

5. Pour over the dressing and mix again.

6. Distribute the salad between two dishes and complete with the shredded chicken. Sprinkle with sesame seeds just before serving.

NUTRITION:

Calories: 345; Fat: 5g; Protein: 4g; Carbohydrates: 10g.

THURSDAY - DAY 25 - DINNER
BUTTERED SALMON

Preparation Time: 10 minutes

Cooking Time: 10 minutes

Servings: 4

INGREDIENTS:

- 4 (5-ounce) skin-on, boneless salmon fillets
- Salt and ground black pepper, to taste
- 1 tablespoon olive oil
- 3 tablespoons butter
- 2 tablespoons lemon juice
- 2 tablespoons fresh rosemary, minced
- 1 teaspoon lemon zest, grated

DIRECTIONS:

1. Season the salmon fillets with salt and black pepper evenly.
2. In a non-stick wok, heat oil over medium heat.
3. Place the salmon fillets, skin side down, and cook for about 3-5 minutes, without stirring.
4. Flip the salmon fillets and cook for about 2 minutes.
5. Add the butter, lemon juice, rosemary, and lemon zest, and cook for about 2 minutes, spooning the butter sauce over the salmon fillets occasionally.
6. Serve hot.

NUTRITION:

Calories: 301; Fat: 21.2g; Protein: 27.7g; Carbohydrates: 1.3g.

FRIDAY - DAY 26 - BREAKFAST
CHEESECAKE CUPS

Preparation Time: 5 minutes

Cooking Time: 0 minutes

Servings: 4 servings

INGREDIENTS:

- 8 ounces cream cheese, softened
- 2 ounces heavy cream
- 1 teaspoon Stevia Glycerite
- 1 teaspoon Splenda
- 1 teaspoon vanilla flavoring (Frontier Organic)

DIRECTIONS:

1. Combine all the ingredients.
2. Whip until a pudding consistency is achieved.
3. Divide into cups.
4. Refrigerate until served!

NUTRITION:

Calories: 205; Fat: 19g; Protein: 5g; Carbohydrates: 2g.

FRIDAY - DAY 26 - LUNCH
TUNA CAKES

Preparation Time: 15 minutes

Cooking Time: 10 minutes

Servings: 2

INGREDIENTS:

- 1 (15-ounce) can water-packed tuna, drained
- ½ celery stalk, chopped
- 2 tablespoons fresh parsley, chopped
- 1 teaspoon fresh dill, chopped
- 2 tablespoons walnuts, chopped
- 2 tablespoons mayonnaise
- 1 organic egg, beaten
- 1 tablespoon butter
- 3 cups lettuce

DIRECTIONS:

1. Add all ingredients (except the butter and lettuce) in a bowl and mix until well-combined.
2. Make two equal-sized patties from the mixture.
3. Melt some butter and cook the patties for about 2-3 minutes.
4. Carefully flip the side and cook for about 2-3 minutes.
5. Divide the lettuce onto serving plates.
6. Top each plate with one burger and serve.

NUTRITION:

Calories: 267; Fat: 12.5g; Protein: 11.5g; Carbohydrates: 3.8g.

FRIDAY - DAY 26 - DINNER
GREEK VEGGIE BRIAM

Preparation Time: 10 minutes

Cooking Time: 30 minutes

Servings: 4

INGREDIENTS:

1/3 cup good-quality olive oil, divided

1 onion, thinly sliced

1 tablespoon minced garlic

¾ small eggplant, diced

2 zucchinis, diced

2 cups chopped cauliflower

1 red bell pepper, diced

2 cups diced tomatoes

2 tablespoons chopped fresh parsley

2 tablespoons chopped fresh oregano

Sea salt, for seasoning

Freshly ground black pepper, for seasoning

1 ½ cups crumbled feta cheese

¼ cup pumpkin seeds

DIRECTIONS:

1. Preheat the oven. Set the oven to broil and lightly grease a 9-by-13-inch casserole dish with olive oil.
2. Sauté the aromatics in a medium stockpot over medium heat, warm 3 tablespoons of the olive oil. Add the onion and garlic and sauté until they've softened, about 3 minutes.
3. Sauté the vegetables. Stir in the eggplant, cook, stirring occasionally.
4. Add the zucchini, cauliflower, and red bell pepper and cook for 5 minutes.

5. Stir in the tomatoes, parsley, and oregano and cook, stirring from time to time, until the vegetables are tender, about 10 minutes. Season it with salt and pepper.

6. Broil. Put vegetable mix in the casserole dish and top with the crumbled feta. Broil until the cheese is melted.

7. Serve. Divide the casserole between four plates and top it with the pumpkin seeds. Drizzle with the remaining olive oil.

NUTRITION:

Calories: 341; Fat: 5.1g; Protein: 1.4g; Carbohydrates: 1.2g.

SATURDAY - DAY 27 - BREAKFAST
STRAWBERRY SHAKE

Preparation Time: 5 minutes

Cooking Time: 0 minutes

Servings: 1 serving

INGREDIENTS:

- ¾ cup coconut milk (from the carton)
- ¼ cup heavy cream
- 7 ice cubes
- 2 tablespoons sugar-free strawberry Torani syrup
- ¼ teaspoon Xanthan Gum

DIRECTIONS:

1. Combine all the ingredients into blender.
2. Blend for 1-2 minutes.
3. Serve!

NUTRITION:

Calories: 270; Fat: 27g; Protein: 2.5g; Carbohydrates: 6.5g.

SATURDAY - DAY 27 - LUNCH

PIZZA BIANCA

Preparation Time: 10 minutes

Cooking Time: 10 minutes

Servings: 2

INGREDIENTS:

- 2 tablespoons olive oil
- 4 eggs
- 2 tablespoons water
- 1 jalapeño pepper, diced
- ¼ cup mozzarella cheese, shredded
- 2 chives, chopped
- 2 cups egg Alfredo sauce
- ½ teaspoon oregano
- ½ cup mushrooms, sliced

DIRECTIONS:

1. Preheat oven to 360°F.
2. In a bowl, whisk eggs, water, and oregano. Heat the olive oil in a large skillet.
3. The egg mixture must be poured in, then let it cook until set, flipping once.
4. Remove and spread the Alfredo sauce and jalapeño pepper all over.
5. Top with mozzarella cheese, mushrooms and chives. Let it bake for 10 minutes

NUTRITION:

Calories: 314; Fat: 15.6g; Protein: 10.4g; Carbohydrates: 5.9g.

SATURDAY - DAY 27 - DINNER
ROASTED TENDERLOIN

Preparation Time: 10 minutes

Cooking Time: 50 minutes

Servings: 10

INGREDIENTS:

- 1 grass-fed beef tenderloin roast
- 4 garlic cloves
- 1 tablespoon rosemary
- Salt
- Ground black pepper
- 1 tablespoon olive oil

DIRECTIONS:

1. Warm-up oven to 425°F.
2. Place beef meat into the prepared roasting pan. Massage with garlic, rosemary, salt, and black pepper and oil. Roast the beef for 45-50 minutes.
3. Remove, cool, slice, and serve.

NUTRITION:

Calories: 295; Fat: 13.9g; Protein: 39.5g; Carbohydrates: 0.6g.

SUNDAY - DAY 28 - BREAKFAST
BACON HASH

Preparation Time: 5 minutes

Cooking Time: 10 minutes

Servings: 2

INGREDIENTS:

- 1 small green pepper
- 2 jalapeno peppers
- 1 small onion
- 4 eggs
- 6 bacon slices

DIRECTIONS:

1. Chop the bacon into chunks using a food processor. Set aside for now. Slice the onions and peppers into thin strips. Dice the jalapenos as small as possible.
2. Heat a skillet and fry the veggies. Once browned, combine the ingredients and cook until crispy. Place on a serving dish with fried eggs.

NUTRITION:

Calories: 366; Fat: 24g; Protein: 23g; Carbohydrates: 9g.

SUNDAY - DAY 28 - LUNCH
TEMPURA ZUCCHINI WITH CREAM CHEESE DIP

Preparation Time: 15 minutes

Cooking Time: 15 minutes

Servings: 4

INGREDIENTS:

Tempura zucchinis:

1 ½ cups (200g) almond flour

2 tablespoons heavy cream

1 teaspoon salt

2 tablespoons olive oil + extra for frying

1 ¼ cups (300ml) water

½ tablespoon sugar-free maple syrup

2 large zucchinis, cut into 1-inch thick strips

Cream cheese dip:

8 onces cream cheese, room temperature

½ cup (113g) sour cream

1 teaspoon taco seasoning

1 scallion, chopped

1 green chili, deseeded and minced

DIRECTIONS:

1. In a bowl, mix the almond flour, heavy cream, salt, peanut oil, water, and maple syrup.
2. Dredge the zucchini strips in the mixture until well-coated.
3. Heat about four tablespoons of olive oil in a non-stick skillet.
4. Working in batches, use tongs to remove the zucchinis (draining extra liquid) into the oil.
5. Fry per side for 1 to 2 minutes and remove the zucchinis onto a paper towel-lined plate to drain grease.

6. In a bowl or container, mix the cream cheese, taco seasoning, sour cream, scallion, and green chili.

7. Serve the tempura zucchinis with the cream cheese dip.

NUTRITION:

Calories: 316; Fat: 8.4g; Protein: 5.1g; Carbohydrates: 4.1g.

SUNDAY - DAY 28 - DINNER
CREAMY PARMESAN SHRIMP

Preparation Time: 10 minutes

Cooking Time: 20 minutes

Servings: 4

INGREDIENTS:

1 ½ pounds shrimp

½ cup chicken stock

¼ teaspoon red pepper flakes

1 cup parmesan cheese, grated

1 cup fresh basil leaves

1 ½ cups heavy cream

¼ teaspoon paprika

3 ounces roasted red peppers, sliced

½ onion, minced

1 tablespoon garlic, minced

3 tablespoons butter

Pepper

Salt

DIRECTIONS:

1. Melt 2 tablespoons butter in a pan over medium heat.
2. Season shrimp with pepper and salt and sear in a pan for 1-2 minutes. Transfer shrimp on a plate.
3. Add remaining butter in a pan.
4. Add red chili flakes, paprika, roasted peppers, garlic, onion, pepper, and salt and cook for 5 minutes.
5. Add stock and stir well and cook until liquid reduced by half.

6. Turn heat to low, add cream and stir for 1-2 minutes.
7. Add basil and parmesan cheese and stir for 1-2 minutes.
8. Return shrimp to the pan and cook for 1-2 minutes.
9. Serve and enjoy.

NUTRITION:

Calories: 524; Fat: 33.2g; Protein: 47.8g; Carbohydrates: 8.3g.

MEASUREMENT AND CONVERSIONS

CUPS	OZ	G	TBSP	TSP	ML
1	8	225	16	48	250
3/4	6	170	12	36	175
2/3	5	140	11	32	150
1/2	4	115	8	24	125
1/3	3	70	5	16	70
1/4	2	60	4	12	60
1/8	1	30	2	6	30
1/16	1/2	15	1	3	15
250°F	300°F	325°F	350°F	400°F	450°F
120°C	150°F	160°C	175°C	200°C	230°C

CONCLUSION

Dealing with weight issues can be disheartening, and you do not have to be extremely overweight or obese to feel the effects. These extra pounds can put a strain on your overall health and wellness. They can make you less efficient in your work life and everyday activities. They can take you away from the things you like to do and the places you love to visit. They can make you feel winded and out of breath at the simplest activities. They can take away your joy for living and living life to the fullest.

When people get older, their bones weaken. At 50, your bones are likely not as strong as they used to be; however, you can keep them in really good conditions. Consuming milk to give calcium cannot do enough to strengthen your bones. What you can do is to make use of the Keto diet as it is low in toxins. Toxins negatively affect the absorption of nutrients and so with this, your bones can take in all they need.

Whether you have met your weight loss goals, your life changes, or you simply want to eat whatever you want again. You cannot just suddenly start consuming Carbs again because it will shock your system. Have an idea of what you want to allow back into your consumption slowly. Be familiar with portion sizes and stick to that amount of Carbs for the first few times you eat post-keto.

Start with non-processed Carbs like whole grain, beans, and fruits. Start slow and see how your body reacts before resolving to add Carbs one meal at a time.

The things to watch out for when coming off keto are weight gain, bloating, and feeling hungry. The weight gain is nothing to freak out over; perhaps, you might not even gain any. It all depends on your diet, how your body processes carbs, and, of course, water weight. The length of your keto diet is a significant factor in how much weight you have lost, which is caused by the reduction of Carbs. The bloating will occur because of the reintroduction of fibrous foods and your body getting used to digesting them again. The bloating van lasts for a few days to a few weeks.

The ketogenic diet is the ultimate tool you can use to plan your future. Can you picture being more involved, more productive and efficient, and more relaxed and energetic? That future is possible for you, and it does not have to be a complicated process to achieve that vision. You can choose right now to be healthier and slimmer and more fulfilled tomorrow. It is possible with the ketogenic diet.

This is not a fancy diet that promises falsehoods of miracle weight loss. This diet is proven by years of science and research, which benefits not only your waistline, but your heart, skin, brain, and organs. It does not just improve your physical health but your mental and emotional health as well. This diet improves your health holistically.

Printed in Great Britain
by Amazon